NURSING HOMES

THE COMPLETE GUIDE

NURSING HOMES

THE COMPLETE GUIDE

MARY BRUMBY FORREST, LPN
CHRISTOPHER B. FORREST, M.D.
RICHARD FORREST

TAYLOR PUBLISHING COMPANY

Published by Taylor Publishing Company
1550 West Mockingbird Lane
Dallas, Texas 75235

Designed by Ron Monteleone.

Library of Congress Cataloging-in-Publication Data

Forrest, Mary Brumby.
　[Nursing homes]
　The complete nursing home guide : finding quality care for your loved ones / Mary Brumby Forrest, Christopher B. Forrest, Richard Forrest.
　　p.　　cm.
　Originally published: Nursing homes. New York : Facts on File, 1990.
　Includes bibliographical references and index.
　ISBN 0-87833-822-5
　1. Nursing homes.　2. Nursing homes—Evaluation.　I. Forrest, Christopher B.　II. Forrest, Richard.　III. Title.
　RA997.F67　1993
　362.1'6—dc20　　　　　　　　　　　　　　　　　　　92-37175
　　　　　　　　　　　　　　　　　　　　　　　　　　　　　CIP

Printed in the United States of America

10 9 8 7 6 5 4 3 2 1

This is an authorized reprint of *Nursing Homes: The Complete Guide,* first published by Facts on File, Inc. in 1990.

TABLE OF
CONTENTS

ACKNOWLEDGMENTS

The authors are completely responsible for all conclusions and opinions in this book unless otherwise specifically stated. However, the range of subject matter is so vast that we were dependent upon countless others for help and direction. It is impossible to list all the helpful telephone conversations, and the often confidential conversations with patients and staff members we had in skilled nursing homes.

We would like to recognize the following busy individuals who took hours of their time to share their knowledge with us:

John Abbot, Connecticut Hospice; Andrew M. Berliner, D.P.M., Podiatrist; Deborah Brody, Editor; Katherine Forrest, Attorney; Christine Francese, Nursing Home Administrator; Howard Frumkin, M.D.; Joseph Fuller, M.D.; Louis Halprin, Executive Secretary professional organization; Christopher Kriter, Administrator of Life Care Facility; D. Leonard Lieberman Jr., PHD., Nursing Home Administrator; Susan L. Sandel, PHD., Nursing Home Administrator; James Sbrolla, Nursing Home Administrator; William Schwartz, M.D.; Michael Spada, Board and Care Administrator; Christine Sypher, R.N., C., D.N.S., Director of Nursing; Phyllis Westberg, Agent; Eillen Winchell, R.N., Discharge Planner.

*For the nursing home residents,
their families,
and the nurses and aides who care for them.*

NURSING HOMES

THE COMPLETE GUIDE

INTRODUCTION

In our collective minds there are certain words that conjure feelings of dread, distaste and even fear. **Nursing homes are two of those words.**

It would be a gross understatement to say that the nursing home industry has had a bad press. The unfavorable news stories, magazine articles and television exposés on this topic are legion. Their number make acid rain, depletion of the rain forests and holes in the ozone layer appear nearly beneficial. Unlike these other issues, nursing homes make many of us uncomfortable because we don't live in a rain forest, can't tell acid from regular rain and think ozone layers are somewhere up near the North Pole. But, we know that we, our parents or at least a good friend might be forced into a nursing home. The odds are good that we are going to have to deal with this unpleasant topic at some near or far juncture, and we don't like the prospect.

There are good nursing homes. They offer intelligent, skilled and compassionate care to their residents. These facilities are not only medically necessary, but often provide a desirable alternative to other types of living situations.

There are nursing homes which should be avoided at all cost. These facilities provide such poor care and undesirable quality of life that the morbidity and mortality rates of their patients increase in an alarming manner. In 1989 state investigators from the New York State Department of Health found a nursing home where 68% of the patients were restrained, 36% had contractures (permanent stiffening of the joints) and 13% had bedsores. They also concluded that this nursing home did not meet state standards for resident rights, infection control, nutrition, nursing services, administration of drugs and patient care management.

This book will provide the criteria for finding the good nursing homes and avoiding the bad nursing homes. Since this is a "complete guide," it will attempt far more than that, but if it keeps one person from spending one day in such a place as described above, it will have succeeded.

1

A MYTH

There is a myth in the American psyche that evokes a past perfection. This legend is composed of elm–shaded streets that are lined with comfortable homes fronted with wide porches filled with high wicker chairs and slatted swings swaying gently on their chains. An occasional iron deer is poised proudly on a neatly trimmed front lawn. Every house is home to a large multi–generational family. Each morning Father leaves for work, resplendent in a starched shirt with Celluloid collar. He walks a few blocks to the trolley line with a newspaper neatly folded under his arm. Mother spends the morning baking fresh bread, and her afternoons are busy with volunteer work in one of her many charities. Obedient children hurry to school where they are sternly taught the basics.

Grandmother lives comfortably in a sun–splashed bedroom on the first floor that is filled with her memorabilia of a productive life. She is a vision of sweetness and gentility, and her sage wisdom and placid personality are the keystones of family solidarity. At an advanced age Grandmother becomes ill with a painless but weakening disease of vague origin.

The loyal family doctor, who seems to resemble Robert Young, spends countless hours at her bedside before announcing solemnly to the family that, "She is leaving us now."

The family's solicitude is boundless as they surround the deathbed. They are rewarded with a few parting gestures of love and advice as Grandmother passes from this vale surrounded by her adoring and grieving family.

For the moment, let us disregard how hard those Victorian barns were to heat. Let us put aside how many hours a day Mother toiled at tedious household chores, or the 60 hours a week that Father worked. We will forget that although the kids may have been taught basics, few of them finished high school. Let us realistically consider Grandmother in the front bedroom.

Our 1900 grandmother simply wasn't there. If she were one of the few, who through chance or heredity reached 60, she probably died during the first difficult winter from pneumonia or influenza.

LIFE EXPECTANCY

Life expectancy in 1900 was 47. Only 4% of the population reached 65. If this sounds bleak, remember that in ancient Greece you lived to 18; in 1600 you lived to a ripe old 33; and you were a senior citizen at 40 during the Civil War.

Since the turn of the century, life expectancy has increased 28 years, and

FIG. 1: LIFE EXPECTANCY FROM 1950–1990

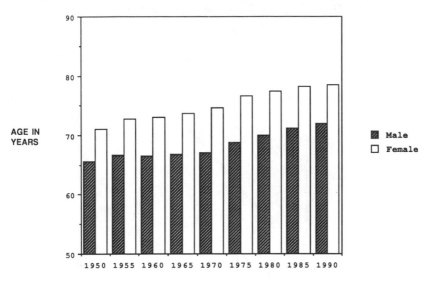

Source: U.S. National Center for Health Statistics

is now over 75. Two-thirds of mankind's increase in life span since prehistory has taken place during the last 50 years.

In 1950 a man in the United States could expect to live 65.6 years and a woman 71.1 years. The projected life expectancies for men and women in 1990 are 72 and 78.5 years respectively (see Figure 1).

During this same 40 year period, Americans over the age of 65 have doubled so that they now number over 28.5 million or 12% of the population.

The older population grows older. The 75–84 age group is 11 times larger than it was in 1900, while the 85+ group is 22 times larger. Figure 2 shows past and projected figures from the Census Bureau for the 85+ group and demonstrates that the size of this segment of the U.S. population will continue to escalate. By the year 2060 there will be five times as many people over 85 as there were in 1940.

The major part of this increase in life expectancy occurred because of reduced death rates for children and young adults due to improved sanitation, decreased crowding, vaccinations and better nutrition. The longevity of the elderly has increased due to an explosion of knowledge in medical science during the past 50 years. A few decades ago pneumonia was considered the ''great remover'' of the elderly. It was a common disease, and its onset was a virtual death sentence. Today, a host of effective antibiotics and other drugs can control, cure or mitigate the effects of countless afflic-

FIG. 2: CUMULATIVE PERCENTAGE INCREASE IN THE UNITED STATES OF PEOPLE OVER 85, 1940–2060.

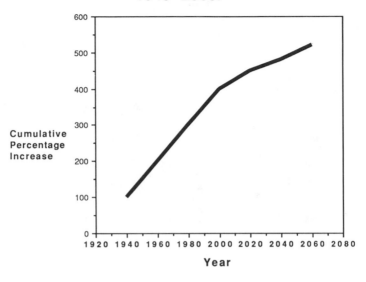

tions that would have been deadly in the past. Improved anesthesia and surgical techniques have made operations routine for individuals in their 70s, 80s and even 90s.

WHO ARE THE ELDERLY? AND HOW DID THEY GET THAT WAY?

Over 50 years ago when social security was established and pension plans began to flourish, the age of 65 was arbitrarily selected as the time of retirement. It seemed to make sense then, but increased longevity due to changes in life–style and the march of medical progress has tilted this arbitrary demarcation point in a skewed fashion.

Alzheimer's disease can strike individuals in their 40s, while 70 year-olds occasionally run the Boston Marathon. Progeria, a rare childhood disease, causes premature aging and affected individuals die in their teens. We know of nursing home patients in their 60s, and octogenarians living full lives in their own apartments. For some, aging seems to cease somewhere in their middle 60s and they continue into their late 80s without apparent change, while others of us seem old before our time.

Although social security and many retirement plans may be based on the still arbitrary age of 65, "old age" or "the elderly" is usually defined as those over 75. Those elderly with one or more medical conditions that inhibit full function have been termed the "frail elderly." Longevity, or the longest life span possible, is marked at 115 years for humans; while life expectancy, the life span for the average person, is now calculated at the mid–70s and will probably plateau at 85 in the future.

Webster's Ninth New Collegiate Dictionary defines aging as, "to become old, to show the effects or the characteristics of increasing age." Aging is defined by the 22nd edition of *Dorland's Medical Dictionary* as, "the gradual structural changes that occur with the passage of time, that are not due to accident or disease, and that eventually lead to increased probability of death as the organism grows older."

These definitions are circular, for they seem to say that we age because we get older—which really doesn't tell us very much. What we do know is that growing older brings certain physical changes as normal aspects of aging. These may be discomforting and even disconcerting, but they are not necessarily incapacitating. As we age we have less endurance, our reaction time and our agility slow and we tire more easily. The female looses capacity to bear children after menopause, and both sexes may have a loss of hearing in the higher tones, less visual acuity and more brittle bones. There is no loss of cognitive functions as part of aging, although we may be less plastic in our response to environmental changes. Some intellectual functions, such as word usage, actually increase with age.

At the turn of the century, the Russian zoologist and bacteriologist Elie Metchnikoff theorized that noxious bacteria flourished in our systems and produced toxins that ultimately killed us. In the 1920s research focused on endocrine glands, and in the 1950s one theory held that random biological damage eventually accumulated to a lethal dose.

In 1920 an American, Raymond Pearl, performed an aging study which resulted in what to us now is not a remarkable conclusion: Individuals with grandparents who lived long tend to have long life spans. This was the first scientific study to imply that aging may have an inherited (i.e., genetic) component.

Modern scientific theory seems to hold that there is some sort of programmed aging built into our genes. The life span of identical twins, two individuals with the same genes, is closer than that of fraternal twins or siblings. Descendants of centenarians, when compared to a group of people with ancestors of average life span, live longer. In general, life expectancy of any individual is best gauged by family history. You live about as long as your family.

The body continuously replaces worn–out cells by the millions each day of our lives. As the years pass, this rate of replacement slows down very gradually. It is so gradual that between the years of 40 and 60 it is hardly noticible. The process of aging may be hastened by environmental conditions, disease, emotional stress or nutrition.

In the early 1960s Leonard Hayflick provided solid experimental evidence for a genetically determined aging process. He observed that certain types of skin cells that grow well in a petri dish have a limited number of times they replicate. They seem to die after 50 divisions. The same types of cells from older individuals and individuals with diabetes, a medical condition which is known to accelerate the progress of age–related disease, divide fewer times than those of younger people. Hayflick feels that some inherent mechanism must exist in the cell which flips on the aging switch. The exact nature of this switch is presently unknown.

The immunologic theory of aging is based upon changes in the immune system observed in the elderly. Older people have a diminished ability to produce antibodies, infection fighting proteins, which are found in the blood and produced by white blood cells. The immune system becomes less able to distinguish between what is part of the body and what is foreign, such as bacteria. As a consequence of this immune confusion, the amount of autoimmune diseases, a disorder in which the body actually destroys itself, increases. Examples of autoimmune diseases include rheumatoid arthritis, thyroid disease, and adult–onset diabetes. These factors enhance a person's susceptibility to infection and chronic disease including cancer.

There are several points which argue against this theory as a complete explanation of aging. One argument is that many lower animals lack the elaborate immune system of humans, and yet still undergo aging. An increased amount of autoimmune disease may simply be a consequence of a changing body; aging produces changes which baffle the immune system.

Today, despite millions of words in scholarly journals, hundreds of scientists working on the problem and a few novel theories, the answer to why we age is still unknown. A consensus opinion is probably that the answer lies hidden in DNA. This would fit with theories postulating that aging is a result of evolutionary pressure which exerts its effects on DNA templates. Some form of genetically programmed mechanism for aging seems most likely. A genetic program would account for differences in inter–species longevity, and also human family histories of long life spans. Other physiologic effects (such as changes in the immune system) would be secondary to an inherited program. A tremendous amount of research is oriented toward molecular mechanisms of aging and genetic programs.

THE COST OF PROLONGED LIFE

Nearly 50% of those over 65 will have a stay in a nursing home. Twenty–five percent of those over 85 will live in a nursing home.

The dramatic increase in life expectancy has carried a heavy societal financial burden, and often great emotional stress on individuals. As the elderly survive longer, they are often faced with one or more chronic medical conditions requiring care that they and their family are not able to provide. An example of this is Alzheimer's disease.

Only a few years ago this affliction was defined as a presenile dementia that usually had an onset at middle age. As people began to live longer, we began to see more cases in the elderly. We now understand that as many as 2.5 million Americans suffer from Alzheimer's disease, and for those over 80 there is a 20% chance of its occurrence.

As spouses and other family members struggle with this disease they are nearly overwhelmed with the caretaking responsibilities. As the disease progresses, home care usually becomes impossible and institutional placement must be arranged. This stay may last for years, at great cost to families or governmental agencies.

It is not only the financial costs of health care for the aged that are important, but also the emotional trauma as difficult choices are made for alternative life–styles.

In order to provide alternatives for the growing numbers of our elderly, there has been explosive growth in the nursing home industry. However, there are other factors which also must be noted in order to understand the reasons for this astounding increase in nursing home facilities:

1. Congressional passage of the 1965 Older Americans Act not only provided for Medicare, but created a state–federal partnership in Medicaid. Medicaid (called Medi–Cal in California) funds pay for nearly 50% of all nursing home patients. This attracted many profit–making corporations into the field.

2. Recent attempts to curtail acute care hospital costs have focused on shortening inpatient stays. Hosptials have been encouraged—in fact penalized if they did not—to release patients to home care or nursing home care when acute care was not medically indicated.

3. With a national divorce rate of 50%, and the subsequent growth of serial families, combined with the need and desire for women to have careers, there are fewer families with full–time care givers available in the home.

4. Although home care for the elderly is less expensive than a nursing home, the proper mix of skilled and custodial home care is often not available.

5. Our mobile society without the past constraints of church and community has changed perceptions of family duty. Today's family is more apt to consider the quality of life for all members of the family rather than one individual, and therefore is less willing to make disruptive family accommodations.

NURSING HOME FEARS

"Promise me that you won't ever send me to one of those homes!"

How tempting it is to answer this plea with a quick social lie. How easy it is to make the promise, to ignore the realities of a situation, and to respond from the heart. How can we forget the years of marriage? Can we ignore our parents who brought us into this world?

We may ignore the facts that our marriage was less than blessed, that the tension between father and son kept them estranged, or that mother has now become impossible to handle. Even if we were objective, can we still sentence a family member to one of those places? If we do, what happens when it's our turn?

There are few decisions in life that are more difficult or emotionally wrenching than placing someone in a nursing home. The very word, "home," evokes Dickensian specters. We envision gloomy buildings with dark halls and a leaking roof.

We think these places are staffed by sadistic aides who abuse the elderly on the few occasions when they are actually in their presence. The staff makes their rounds on roller skates in order to speed their way back to the lounge where they drink whiskey and when not asleep, bawdily discuss their love lives.

The establishment is presided over by a greedy owner whose lust for profit is insatiable. His rapacious appetite for money keeps him constantly busy in his quest to purchase even cheaper cuts of meat, further reduce the staff and completely do away with the laundry service. When not engaged in those activities, he is involved in the ongoing battle to circumvent governmental regulations or creating new accounting methods to increase patient billings.

And yet, half of us who reach 65 will spend some time in one of those places!

Contrary to the bleak picture portrayed above, the modern nursing home is not an annex to a medieval torture chamber. There are many homes that are light and airy in appearance, provide excellent skilled nursing care and are staffed by dedicated people who not only care, but actually love their residents. There are also nursing homes which have attractive exteriors, well-appointed interiors and yet for any number of reasons do not deliver good patient care. There are also homes that resemble the hypothetical nightmarish situation portrayed above.

The Search

Some of us will have the physical and mental vitality to investigate, research and visit nursing homes in order to make an intelligent decision. Others will act as advocates and perform this function for spouses, parents or friends. Many of us will be discharged from an acute care (general) hospital for a condition that is temporarily incapacitating, but which will only require a short–term nursing home confinement. The new diagnosis related grouping (DRG) rules which the federal government uses for hospital reimbursement has converted many hospital stays into revolving door confinements. This early release often means the necessity for nursing home care after hospital discharge. In such instances, the time available to select a convalescent facility is greatly curtailed.

Unless you have visited nursing homes and have some experience with them, your initial exposure is likely to be overwhelming. Patients use various types of ambulation devices to walk the halls. Some are restrained in wheelchairs, while others speak in gibberish. At the same time, other residents will play chess, read the newest novel or discuss current events in an animated manner. Even in the best of facilities, there is often the faint odor of urine or feces and the mutterings of confused patients.

And from this initial exposure you are expected to make a deicison that will establish the future quality of life for yourself or a loved one.

In most cases the decision to enter a nursing home and the selection of the facility is not made by the resident alone. Due to chronic disabilities often suffered by the elderly which render them frail, or the nature of an acute care hospital stay, the future resident is often removed at least partly from the decision making process.

This book, therefore, must be directed not only to the future resident, but to the family or friends of the potential patient. An exception to this is in the area of life care facilities. These increasingly popular retirement villages offer on–site nursing homes or maintain an arrangement with a nearby nursing home for use by its residents. Individuals selecting this type of alternative living arrangement are not only choosing retirement housing, but selecting a nursing home for possible use in the future.

The Book's Mission

This book provides guidelines that will aid in making the nursing home decision. It explains how to evaluate and choose the proper facility.

It examines the cost of such services, Medicare and Medicaid, long–term care insurance and other important financial data concerning the nursing home resident and family.

Monitoring the patient's nursing care and quality of life are important considerations that are explored, along with helpful hints on admission procedures, prior preparation and visiting.

In addition to the major thrust of the book, it will also consider related topics of profound interest to potential residents and their advocates:

A survey of common geriatric disorders and the nursing care they require will be an important topic.

Chapters will consider the confused patient, senile dementia and the proper use of physical and chemical restraints for those patients.

The family's emotional dynamics as they affect the nursing home decision, visits and other aspects of the patient's life will be explored.

Death in the nursing home, the hospice or at home will be discussed. Consideration will be given to heroic medical measures, living wills, benign neglect of the terminally ill and attitudes toward death by staff and family members.

The material in this book is directed toward facilities that care for the elderly. It does not attempt to measure standards of care for institutions that are involved completely with psychiatric patients, the mentally retarded or units concerned exclusively with rehabilitation programs.

The emphasis has been directed toward the skilled nursing home for it is in this setting that the frailest and most vulnerable residents are domiciled. Nursing homes vary in the amount and complexity of nursing services they offer. They range in type from small rest homes that are primarily custodial in nature, up to those that provide around–the–clock nursing care. The patient in this latter facility, the skilled nursing home, is the least articulate, the least mobile and the most likely to have chronic medical problems. It is those individuals who can suffer the most. Therefore, the book's recommendations are directed toward those facilities, although the majority of the general criteria are valid for any licensed nursing home institution.

CHAPTER 1

PEOPLE WE HAVE KNOWN

CASE HISTORIES OF NURSING HOME PLACEMENTS WITH ANALYSIS

GEORGIA R., 85
AN INCORRECT PLACEMENT

Georgia R. was still a laugher. This was a lifelong trait as faded photographs taken at ancient family outings revealed. It was her smile which always dominated the tableaux, and, after the natural adversities of a long life, her smile and infectious laugh still spilled forth at the slightest provocation.

Widowed for 10 years, Georgia lived with her youngest son, his wife and their three teenage children in a large home on the Connecticut shore. Although free from severe chronic physical complaints, she suffered from high blood pressure (hypertension), difficulty in walking and occasional short-term memory loss. Her physician was concerned over her failure to keep to her prescribed medical regimen. The family was dismayed over her urinary incontinence and her recent lack of personal hygiene.

The family held secret conferences without Georgia and made arrangements for her admission to a nursing home.

ANALYSIS

Georgia's incontinence may be correctable. It is possible that her physician prescribed a diuretic that lowers blood pressure. However, these drugs typically cause frequent urination, and because of her difficulty in walking,

11

Georgia often could not get to the bathroom in time. In order to maintain her dignity, Georgia may have "forgotten" to take her medication.

Incontinence was distressing this family, and is the most widely cited single factor given as a reason for nursing home placement.

If Georgia's incontinence were not due to drugs, the family physician may test her urine for a bladder infection. Other treatable causes of incontinence could be investigated by a urologist, a surgeon with particular expertise in urinary problems. There are also bladder retraining programs.

Georgia may have had a series of transient ischemic attack (TIAs) or small strokes which caused a certain amount of short–term memory loss. It is also possible that her memory lapses were benign forgetfulness, which is common in the elderly. A full workup at a geriatric assessment unit would have been useful to establish clearly the extent of her problems.

Georgia's lack of personal hygiene was due to her realistic assessment of her own physical limitations. She was terrified of falling in the bathroom, and the tub was not equipped with grab bars or a shower stool. She was born near the turn of the century, and had the modesty of that era. She was reluctant to ask members of the family to aid her in bathing. She refused to bathe not because of senility, but because of normal fears and feelings.

The family's secret decision to place her in a nursing home made her acclimation doubly difficult. She felt abandoned and resentful. It is common for alert nursing home residents who are not a part of the decision making process to have strong feelings of resentment at their situation. In one dramatic incident, an alert elderly man was taken for a "ride in the country" and left at a nursing home while the family fled. The physical, emotional and intellectual capacity of this patient was immediately altered.

The gradual loss of control over one's life is one of the most depressing aspects of growing old. Involuntary confinement to a nursing home is the ultimate loss of control.

The results of Georgia's placement were disastrous. The family, torn with guilt, vacillated between visiting her haphazardly and visiting excessively in a disruptive manner that made acclimation even more difficult. Georgia was not happy, her quality of life declined and she lost her laughter.

And yet . . .

Georgia was already part of a family unit that had adjusted to her pleasant presence under normal circumstances. Her health care needs were minimal, and if the family had turned to outside sources for aid, most of the problems could have been solved to everyone's satisfaction.

The local Visiting Nurse Service or Home Health Care Agency could have been contacted to arrange for regular visits to help Georgia bathe and to encourage her adherence to the medical regimen. Her physician might have prescribed an alternative drug for her hypertension that did not cause diuresis. A urologist may have been consulted, and if all else failed, special clothing and pads could have mitigated the problem of incontinence. Proper grab bars, rubber mats and a stool should have been installed in the bathroom.

With such minimal care and consideration, Georgia could have continued living at home for an indefinite period.

WILLIAM T., 68
A TRANSFER FROM AN ACUTE CARE HOSPITAL

William T. suffered a stroke on the golf course near the sand bunkers just before the fourth green. He was preparing for an easy chip shot when he felt a rush of weakness which was quickly followed by nausea and dizziness. He stopped stock–still and felt the tendrils of pain from a severe headache.

In less than 30 minutes the ambulance delivered him to the emergency room of the local hospital. Wiliam was diagnosed as having suffered a cerebrovascular accident (CVA), also known as a stroke, shock or apoplexy. CVA stands in third place behind heart disease and cancer as a leading cause of death in the elderly, but 75% of its victims can learn to ambulate, and over 15% will return to work or independent life.

William suffered from right sided weakness which meant he had a left sided CVA. This affected is ability to communicate. If he had left sided weakness, signifying a right sided CVA, communication might not have been impaired.

William's attending physician and the hospital administration will feel pressure to discharge him promptly. Recent regulations by the federal government administered through Medicare financially penalize hospitals if they do not discharge patients when acute hospital care is not needed. But, many of these patients are not ready or able to participate in home care at that time!

William needed skilled nursing care for further stabilization and physical rehabilitation along with speech and occupational therapy. It was necessary to reteach him some of the basic functions of life such as shaving, dressing and other activities of daily living.

In William's case, the family had no nursing home preference and he was transferred to a facility selected by the hospital's discharge planner.

ANALYSIS

As required, the hospital's discharge planner chose a nursing home that was Medicare–approved, since that insurance would pay part of the costs in this instance. A Medicare–approved home would adhere to at least basic governmental standards, but the discharge planner is under no directive to select a nursing home by any other criteria. The facility selected may or may not have been appropriate for William's urgent physical and psychological needs.

Stroke patients are often depressed. Aphasic stroke patients are always depressed, despondent and often agitated. It is important to realize that the inability to communicate does not necessarily mean there is a loss of mental competence. Recovery from these symptoms is typically lengthy. Attitude is one of the single most important elements in the stroke patient returning to a normal and independent life.

The outlook of stroke patients can be compared to the emotional stages of the terminally ill. Dr. Elisabeth Kubler–Ross, in her book, *On Death and Dying,* lists these stages as: denial, anger, bargaining, depression, and acceptance, with the persistence of hope throughout. If stroke patients are treated with understanding, they can often work through this emotional labyrinth toward a quality of life only slightly less restricted than their former lives.

In addition to dealing with depression, the stroke patient will require a great deal of time spent in perfecting activities of daily living (ADL). Reteaching ADLs (which includes such normal functions as using a fork or brushing one's hair) is time consuming for the nursing home staff. It is easier for the nurse or aide to perform these tasks for the patient rather than stand impatiently nearby while the patient struggles with what are now difficult movements. Harried staff members with high patient loads, or even well–meaning family members, will often take the easy way out and "help" the patient with these ADLs. This "help" increases the patient's sense of dependency and inhibits recovery.

It is impossible to say that nursing care for one category of patient is more important than another, but the need for quality care is dramatically obvious in stroke cases. It is common to see stroke victims of similar age, medical background and degree of impairment recover at radically different rates. While one patient will make rapid positive strides and return home to an independent life, another might "turn to the wall" and become increasingly dependent, bitter and show few signs of recovery.

William's acute medical problem needed stabilization, and he required intelligent nursing care for his psychological problems. He required good physical, occupational and speech therapy, with a staff that would emphasize his relearning the activities of daily living.

How apparent it is that the quality of his nursing home would be a critical factor in his full recovery.

HATTIE L., 72
SENILE DEMENTIA, ALZHEIMER'S TYPE

Hattie L., a widow, was physically unimpaired, and until some months ago, led a full and independent life.

Since her childhood school days, Hattie had always been a list maker. This habit was helpful in her aggressive volunteer activities with the local chapter of the Red Cross. She was often in charge of their annual fund–raising effort, and her lists were filled with names and appointments.

Then she forgot to make note of appointments or completely misplaced her list. She began to forget where she had parked her car during her shopping excursions. On the evening of the annual Red Cross fund–raising dinner, where she was to speak, Hattie left home early but never arrived at the restaurant. At 3:00 A.M. her divorced daughter received a phone call from a distant police department. Hattie had been stopped for a minor traffic violation, but her confusion was so obvious that she had been brought to the police station. She had no knowledge of the dinner she was to have attended, or how she had driven over a hundred miles.

Hattie's daughter moved into the house and continued her teaching career while overseeing the household. Red Cross officials eased Hattie from any position of responsibility in the organization. Her driver's license was surrendered, although Hattie forgot this and continued to drive downtown until her daughter appropriated her car keys.

For a time friends still called on Hattie. Her social graces were so ingrained that she was able to talk in wide generalities, and was often able to hide from her visitors the widening gaps in her memory. Her daughter became aware of the worsening situation when her mother turned to her in complete confusion after an old friend's departure and asked, "Who was that?"

It became obvious that Hattie was unable to continue watching after her own financial affairs. She would often pay one bill several times while forgetting others. Her daughter took control of the checkbook when the lights were turned off for nonpayment.

Hattie began to wander. While her daughter was at work she would often leave the house either partially dressed, or bizarrely dressed. She would walk the streets in aimless patterns, motivated by inner memory patterns that were often decades in the past.

The family physician began to run tests on Hattie. The tests were negative for any pathological condition which might cause her extreme memory loss.

The daughter hired a companion to stay with Hattie during the day. The companion reported to the daughter and a married son who lived in a distant city that Hattie was a "pussy cat" and tended to nap most of the day.

Hattie's time sense had tilted and night had turned into day. It was common for her to attempt to cook breakfast at midnight, or to insist on a trip to the Red Cross at 3:00 A.M. Her daughter began to grow haggard from loss of sleep as she fought to control or at least monitor her mother's nightly activities.

After observing Hattie's behavior, and in the absence of other pathological conditions, the family physician diagnosed Hattie as having senile dementia, Alzheimer's type.

Hattie began to become increasingly agitated when she was restrained from bizarre activities. Her day companions quit when they were struck while attempting to reason with Hattie or restrain her.

Hattie's daughter took a leave of absence from her teaching job in order to devote herself full–time to the care of her mother. She found that there weren't enough hours in the day. While she performed routine household chores and errands, her mother slept. When she attempted to sleep, her mother prowled. She reached the point of utter mental and physical exhaustion when her mother failed to recognize her, and often slapped her out of frustration.

Hattie's daughter called her brother long distance and informed him that their mother had to go to a home.

"Our mother will never go into one of those places," he categorically announced.

"Then I'll go into one," she replied. "I can't take it anymore."

ANALYSIS

Two and a half million Americans suffer from Alzheimer's disease. Its diagnosis is by exclusion, which is to say that all other possibilities have been considered. In order to shorten this potentially lengthy process, geriatric assessment centers, found at large metropolitan hospitals, are recommended for elderly patients exhibiting profound confusion.

Hattie had progressed through stage one of the disease, impaired short–term memory. She began to exhibit the classic symptoms of stage two: time distortion, profound memory loss, agitation and hostility. As the disease progresses, she will have further memory loss until she will not recognize her children or be able to perform basic social functions. Her distortion of time and memory requires that she be monitored on a 24–hour basis.

An insidious pendulum clock ticks with a double stroke within Hattie. On one sweep there is the irregular but irrevocable progression of the disease. Medical science cannot predict, in any given case, how rapidly a patient will slide from one plateau to another. The only general rule is that an early onset is associated with rapid disease progression.

The back sweep of Hattie's internal clock pertains to her inner sense of time. She might awaken at 3:00 A.M. on any given night intent on either going to a Red Cross fund–raising, or to her sixth grade class picnic. There is no predictability of what era in her past she might enter at any given moment, only that an inexorable slide backward into the earlier reaches of memory will continue.

Hattie's family lives with a clock of their own. In this case as in so many others her daughter is the primary caregiver ("sister care" or care by a female family member). The daughter, at her brother's insistence, may be forced to put her own career permanently in abeyance, and call upon community resources for day care, respite care and support groups. She may manage to keep her mother at home until the next profound stage of the disease.

Unless Hattie should succumb to an acute illness, the question is not IF she will go to a nursing home, the question is WHEN!

The final nursing home placement decision will probably be made in haste when the situation has reached crisis proportions. The crisis will occur either when the daughter is physically and emotionally unable to continue her care giving, or Hattie's behavior becomes intolerable and dangerous to herself and others or, as so often happens, a combination of both circumstances.

WICKED WITCH OF THE WEST, 80
A COMPOSITE OF SEVERAL WITCHES WE HAVE KNOWN

Even witches have children and grow old. The Wicked Witch of the West, known unaffectionally as WWW, seemed to have had every affliction known to mankind, including several that had been eradicated by medical science. She had run through every medical practitioner in the medium–sized city where she lived, and was usually the first patient of any new doctor. She often "took to the bed," although remarkable recoveries were observed if the motivation was adequate. She was often incontinent because she knew that this "really got" the family member entrusted with her care for that day.

WWW's subspecialty, after loudly voicing symptoms, was her transmission of that virulent virus, "the guilt trip." She had honed this ability to a state of the art perfection, and could reduce younger members of the family to tears in minutes, while more experienced adults often took as long as an hour.

The guilt trip was usually introduced into conversation by the use of one of several stock phrases: "Don't worry about me, just let me stare at the ceiling all day . . . How I sacrificed for you children . . . I know I am a burden; just give me a pill and let me die . . . No one loves me, and if I'm lucky, God will take me tonight . . . "

Even hypochondriacs become ill, although discovering WWW's true symptoms among the deluge is difficult. Occasionally these patients will inadvertently help by presenting a real symptom that can be objectively measured by a machine or lab test.

Homecare for WWW is impossible. The simple act of fluffing her pillow properly has reduced nurses of 20 years experience to nervous wrecks. Nursing personnel brought into the home soon find themselves accused of misdemeanors, high crimes and treason. They are summarily fired or else quickly leave to join the foreign legion.

Family members are required by WWW, for it is only with the clan that she can continue her manipulations. Large families, with 10 or more siblings who draw straws for this duty on a regular basis, have been known to provide home care for WWW for as long as a month. After several divorces, a case of alcoholism and a mental hospital admission or two, a family conference votes WWW into the home.

ANALYSIS

The old do not grow sweet in direct proportion to their advancing years. WWW was a brat at 10, a bitch at 20, a witch at 40 and impossible at 80. Her children and grandchildren do not like her very much. This sublimated feeling festers, because everyone knows, "you're supposed to love your mother." When WWW is transported to the nursing home, this family guilt will play havoc with the staff and administrators of the institution. The family will attempt to expiate their guilt by frequent complaints to the staff (after all, they have learned this from a master teacher). Their constant complaints will be fueled under WWW's direction.

Granted that WWW is a composite, but the underlying facts and dynamics are often seen. WWW's magnification of her physical symptoms was due to her increasing awareness of the frailty of her body. Her guilt virus is an awkward attempt for attention and love. She does not want strangers caring for her because she cannot abuse them in the same manner as her family. In a skewed sense, this abuse is an attempt to build a love bridge across the generations in the only way she knows. People who have suffered from love and communication defects throughout their lives will have these defects exaggerated as they age and the covering mask of social graces peels away.

LAWRENCE F., 90
AN IMPOSSIBLE HOME CARE SITUATION

Lawrence was bedridden due to a hip injury suffered in a fall over a year ago. Corrective surgery might help the defect, but the attending physician advised against surgery due to Lawrence's congestive heart failure, emphysema and recent urinary tract infection. Lawrence lived with his son and daughter–in–law.

Incontinence caused by the urinary tract infection and immobility predisposed him to the development of bedsores. The visiting nurse and family doctor recommended that great care be taken to change gowns and bedding after each voiding, and that Lawrence be turned every two hours as an aid to healing the bedsores. A home care nurse was hired for two hours a day to provide treatments and other nursing care for the patient. Due to the nature of the case, the remainder of the care fell on Mary, the daughter–in–law.

Lawrence's son and his wife are in their late 60s, and the case was exacerbated because of the son's heart condition which also required Mary's time. Mary quickly became exhausted as she ran from one bedroom to another in her attempt to take care of two bedridden individuals.

ANALYSIS

It quickly becomes obvious that Mary could not care for both individuals simultaneously. She would either ruin her own health, provide inadequate care for both men or continue until exhaustion took the decision out of her hands.

This is an example of a situation that is becoming more prevalent as life expectancy increases. The elderly are attempting to care for their seniors, who are even more elderly and frail.

If this family were possessed of unlimited funds, they might hire around–the–clock help for the patients. The cost of this type of home care, most of which is *not* covered by insurance or governmental programs, would run from $1,680 per week to $3,360 per week. In addition to the financial cost of this type of care, in most areas of the country it is difficult to obtain properly trained and reliable individuals for this work.

REBECCA Z., 76
ALONE

Rebecca was a childless widow with no immediate relatives. She suffered from several chronic medical problems: diabetes mellitus, hypertension and severe arthritis. Home health care aides on a part–time basis were not sufficient to meet her needs.

ANALYSIS

Half of all older women are widows. There are five times as many widows as widowers, so Rebecca's situation is not unusual. She is also one of the 41% of elderly women who live alone. Although she was able to obtain adequate day nursing care and homemaker services, as her chronic conditions deteriorated, she needed around–the–clock monitoring. Although she may have wished to remain in her own apartment (many in this type of situation do not), her health needs reached a point where they transcended her desire and required her placement in a nursing home with its constant care capabilities.

PATTERNS
IN NURSING HOME ADMISSIONS

There are several patterns apparent in the cases recounted: the transfer from the acute care hospital, the care of the elderly by the elderly, the chronically ill elderly without relatives to supplement home care and the aging witch who no one could tolerate. In these instances it seemed rather obvious that a nursing home placement was either required, or the best alternative under the circumstances. In the two remaining cases, one, Georgia, did not need to go to a nursing home, and in the instance of the patient with Alzheimer's disease, the question was *when* the decision should have been made.

These case histories were selected because they did have an underlying theme or pattern. However, there are as many variations as there are individuals.

CHAPTER 2

WHEN TO GO

MAKING THE NURSING HOME DECISION

TEN RULES

The nursing home decision is approached from two radically different starting points. For some elderly, the decision is a foregone conclusion. They are to be discharged from an acute care hospital, require transfer from a custodial care nursing home or live at home with major medical problems that require 24–hour nursing care. In these instances the element of choice does not rest with the individual or family: It is a medical necessity. But when the medical need is not absolute, when other arrangements *might* be adequate and when additional sacrifice *may* solve the problem, the decision becomes an emotionally wrenching quandary.

How easy it is to make the placement decision if the patient is bedridden, combative and confused or suffering from an array of chronic medical conditions.

How easy it is to make the decision when we are informed by doctors, nurses and therapists that the patient *must* have skilled nursing care for more than just a few hours a day.

How difficult it is to make the decision when it is forced on us by the stress and burden of caring for an elderly individual at home. How difficult the decision is when we are torn by the guilt associated with placing a family member in an institution.

This chapter provides a framework for those undergoing easy and difficult nursing home placement decisions. The rules are set up in a logical progression, and although one or two might not apply in any given case, the principles should be considered in all cases.

Making the Nursing Home Decision

1. Recognize the danger signs given by elderly people living independently.
2. Make an active decision together.
3. Plan the decision in advance.
4. Do not permit an acute care hospital to assume complete control of the nursing home placement.
5. Obtain a complete understanding of the patient's medical condition and prognosis.
6. Assess medical care needs against available resources.
7. Explore your feelings about the placement.
8. Realize that good nursing homes do exist.
9. Provide support for the person entering a nursing home.
10. Understand that the nursing home placement can be a good decision.

RULE 1: RECOGNIZE THE DANGER SIGNS GIVEN BY ELDERLY PEOPLE LIVING INDEPENDENTLY

Mary T., 85

In her later years, Mary exhibited the same feisty independence which characterized her youth. At the age of 16, poor and alone, she boarded an ocean liner that sailed from Ireland to Boston. Her marriage to Big Jimmy, a street cop in South Boston, seemed an equal match for this ginger–haired diminutive lady, but few doubted who ruled the hearth and raised the five children. Widowed at age 80, she continued life without breaking stride. The large house was sold, part of the profit was providently invested, and the remainder purchased a small condominium in a senior citizen's retirement complex. When poor eyesight forced her to surrender her driver's license and then sell her car, she utilized the complex's van service for her errands.

Over a period of several months her family began to see a gradual change in her behavior. Her hair, which previously was perfectly coifed, was tousled, and her dress was generally in disarray. A clandestine search of her kitchen cabinets and refrigerator revealed only a box of corn flakes and a small carton of milk. The family wondered whether Mary's behavior changes were caused by malnutrition.

Mary became obsessed with money. She was convinced that she was destitute and postponed paying bills, buying food and replacing clothes and personal items.

She began to call her children at odd hours of the night claiming that men were trying to break into her apartment. She seemed to lose orientation to time.

The children asked her to sell the condominium and move in with one of them. She adamantly refused and asserted her right to live an independent life. Her children were reluctantly assuaged by her firm refusals.

Early one morning Mary was found by her youngest daughter. She lay dead at the base of the stairwell, having fallen down a flight of metal stairs and suffered a broken neck.

Mary's children should have taken greater heed of the several warning signals she broadcast to them. She exhibited many of the classic danger signs of the elderly living independently who need help:

1. Marked change in personal appearance
2. Decrease in nutritional status
3. Financial confusion
4. Paranoia, hallucinations, and delusions
5. Falls (Falls are the leading cause of accidental death for people over 75. Seventy percent of all fatal falls in the United States involve people over 65.)

In general, significant changes in physical or mental behavior are danger signs. In Mary's case, she did not maintain a proper diet because of monetary delusions. Her apartment could have been filled with food; hoarding would be an equivalent expression of the same fear. Family members should *be alert for signs of change* and less concerned about the actual manifestations of behavior.

Other danger signals to watch for the independent elderly at risk include the following:

1. **Improper use of drugs.** Prescription drugs may not be purchased because of confusion or cost. Forgetting to take a medicine at the proper time is common, just as taking too much of a drug is a worrisome sign.
2. **Potential fire hazards.** Fire hazards are commonly found in the homes of the independent elderly. In Mary's case, she ate corn flakes, which at least kept her away from the stove. It is not uncommon for the elderly to burn pots due to forgetfulness, or to leave cigarettes burning in exposed locations.
3. **Depression.** An extremely common problem in the elderly, depression can lead to substance abuse with alcohol or pills. Because of decreased rates of breakdown and excretion of alcohol in the elderly, one or two drinks can be sufficient for intoxication. Signs of depression should be monitored closely.
4. **Inappropriate emotional responses.** An exaggerated or lack of proper response to key events might be a consequence of memory loss or

FIG.3: DEMOGRAPHIC COMPOSITION OF ELDERLY PEOPLE LIVING ALONE IN 1987

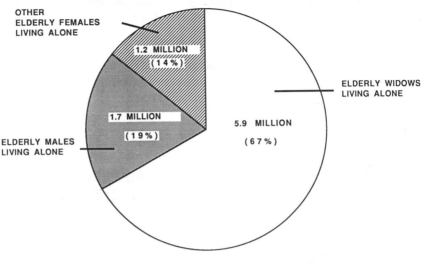

TOTAL = 8.8 MILLION ELDERLY PEOPLE LIVING ALONE

Source: ICF Estimates

confusion and should be considered a danger signal requiring medical assessment.

There are over 8.8 million elderly people living alone (Figure 3), all of whom need monitoring. *Safety must be the prime consideration.* When the integrity of an elderly person's safety cannot be maintained, alternative living arrangements must be made immediately!

RULE 2: MAKE AN ACTIVE DECISION TOGETHER

As we pass through the arch of middle age to the era of old age, there are marked subtractions from our social identity and independence. Retirement from a productive career is one of the most dramatic passages that many face. A great deal of our sense of self–worth is bound to our profession. One day we are responsible employees, and the next pensioners. Many in corporate life or other professions are faced with an arbitrary barrier: age 65. Elderly people find that they are expendable members of a society run for and by the young.

Advancing age is characterized by losses of employment, good health, mobility and independence, reduction of income and the death of friends and spouses. Declining sight and other medical problems often lead to the loss of a driver's license. Houses, often occupied for decades and filled with memories of past life and family, are sold and smaller quarters found. Close friends retire, move away, become ill or die.

All of these late life changes create a sense of isolation in the elderly. The move to a nursing home is therefore perceived as the *ultimate isolation,* and as such may be vigorously resisted.

As we age, our minds become less plastic, and we are less able to cope with changing environments. Due to this, and an unwillingness to cast off the last shreds of identity, the elderly will *resist any change.* This resistance will often manifest itself in many ways if the elderly are asked to consider a nursing home. They do not want to restructure their lives. Often this fear of change will be shrouded by numerous other surface objections which in reality are only a camouflage of the real concern.

The rigid schedule of nursing homes further hampers an elderly person's independence. There is no question that adherence to an institution's rules and regulations is a valid concern and justifiable objection to a placement. *Nursing home regimentation is annoying.* Being told when to get up in the morning and when to go to bed at night smacks of army, prison, academic or parental authority.

If prospective residents are resistant to change, do not welcome nursing home regimentation, and consider this the final isolation, should we wonder why they feel we don't love them? In order to provide the broadest possible emotional support, overcome the patient's natural fears and reservations and allow the smoothest possible transition, *the decision for admission must be mutual.* Inclusion in the decision making process is the best way for the potential resident to overcome feelings of loss and isolation.

Although acute illness or confusion may preclude a mutual dialogue, every effort should be made to include the patient in the decision. In this way you can foster a sense of control over the transfer.

We also recommend that all family members, regardless of location, be sent a written assessment of the nursing home options and the patient's condition. Telephone conversations are convenient, but their results are easily garbled in time's future translations. If brother Henry, living in Point Barrow, Alaska, has suggestions or objections, let him voice them now—not in the future when he has developed perfect hindsight.

It is not suggested that an ill patient be involved in an acrimonious family debate. One primary spokesperson for the family should be selected to talk with the patient and present the consensus of the family deliberations, and attempt to incorporate them within the patient's wishes and desires.

RULE 3: PLAN THE DECISION IN ADVANCE

A forced choice of nursing home under crisis circumstances increases the chance of a poor placement. A short look into the future, be it days, weeks or months, will permit a more thorough and thoughtful investigation of available facilities. **Plan the nursing home placement as far in advance as possible!**

Rule 5 concerns obtaining a complete understanding of the patient's medical condition. Often this information will provide a signal concerning a potential future nursing home placement. Knowing the prognosis of various medical conditions will not allow an exact prediction of when the patient will reach a certain stage, but it will provide rough parameters for planning. Anticipation of when circumstances might require future institutionalization may allow the time necessary for proper planning, searching and family orientation to the problem.

Some placements are obvious (i.e., transfer from another health care facility to a skilled nursing home), others are more nebulous. In some instances the decision is easy because the doctors make it for you.

Doctor T., 72

We moved a stack of medical journals off side chairs and sat before the cluttered desk. Doctor T. signed insurance forms without reading their contents and peered over the rim of his glasses as he spoke with us.

"I did an informal survey of every doc in the county," he said. "Do you know what I found?" He pointed his pen at us to emphasize the point. "The guys who retired only made it for two years, but those of us who kept working are still going strong. Sure, I cut down, and brought a couple of young docs into the practice. I only put in 50 hours a week, these days, but funny, I've gone back to making house calls again."

"Why is that?"

"Hell, some of those people have been patients of mine for over 40 years. They're getting on, they don't go out as much, and some can't drive anymore. Of course, I've got to go to them."

"What advice and counseling do you give your patients and their families concerning the decision to enter a nursing home?"

His gutteral, "Harrumph!" was part laugh and part comment. "I don't counsel or advise. I tell them when to go!"

"And if the patient cannot evaluate your suggestion?"

He tilted his head a moment as he thought about this last remark. "I talk to somebody in the family who's not out to lunch. I find someone, husband, wife, kid, who has still got their marbles, and I tell them it's time. Then I pick up the phone and arrange a bed."

"You make the call after a complete discussion of their financial situation and nursing home preferences?"

He sighed and began signing another stack of forms. "I told you that I've known these people for decades. I know their financial situation. I have privileges at three convalescent hospitals. We call them good, better and best. I call for a bed in the one they can afford."

"And they go?"

"My patients do what I tell them," he said with a note of finality. "Otherwise they wouldn't be my patients. I keep telling that to the young docs in my practice, but they don't seem to get it."

We knew that the young partners he referred to were both in their 40s.

When Doctor T. tells you it's time to go . . . you leave. We also suspect that when this vibrant, elderly doctor arrives in heaven, he'll have a few words with the Maker about the mistakes in the design of the human body. Unfortunately, this type of closely knit doctor–patient relationship is not usual in today's medical practice. Most people will have to seek additional guidance from other sources.

RULE 4: DO NOT PERMIT AN ACUTE CARE HOSPITAL TO ASSUME COMPLETE CONTROL OF THE PLACEMENT

Some individuals will be transferred from an acute care hospital directly to a skilled nursing home for purposes of recuperation, rehabilitation, stabilization or death.

In response to escalating hospital costs, in 1983 Congress passed the Prospective Payment System, a new method of paying hospitals for Medicare and Medicaid. Using information about hospital costs in geographic areas, the government set a standard billing rate for 470 different categories of treatment called diagnosis related groups (DRGs).

DRGs are based on average cost, length of stay in the hospital, medicine charges, physician fees, etc. Thus, if the hospital can incur a lesser charge for hospitalization than that which is reimbursed by a DRG, it will make a profit. For example, a DRG for pneumonia may be based on a seven day hospital stay, but if the patient is discharged after only three days, a profit is made.

DRGs therefore have a built–in incentive for early discharge. Patients are released from the hospital sicker than in the past. In many instances there is a need for skilled nursing care and a transfer to a nursing home. We suggest discussing with the attending physician at the time of admission the expected disposition of the patient after the hospitalization. Forewarned, one might have the opportunity to choose a nursing home rather than accepting an assignment on an available bed basis.

HOSPITAL DISCHARGE PLANNING

Many acute care hospitals employ **discharge planners,** usually social workers or nurses, who work with the hospital staff to determine the level of support needed after discharge. These planners attempt to assess the determined need against available services in the community and resources in the family. When need exceeds resources, a nursing home search is undertaken. For most patients, this balance can be determined shortly after admission. For instance, an elderly person admitted for a broken hip would require seven to 14 days in an acute care hospital and then a longer period of rehabilitation in a nursing home. This common situation lends itself to expeditious discharge planning soon after admission.

Early in the admission the discharge planner should meet with the patient and/or family to initiate planning. Nursing home preferences are honored when possible, but if a choice is not expressed, then the name of the patient will be placed on a revolving first–bed–available list. In New York State, for example, the hospital has the right to place the name of a patient on five waiting lists within a 50 mile radius.

The hospital has no responsibility to check on the quality of the nursing home other than to assure that it is appropriately licensed. Discharge planners are concerned over which homes have available beds and which nursing homes will accept Medicaid patients.

There is no question that the hospital and the patient can develop an adversarial relationship while disposition is decided. When the DRG time allotment has expired, the hospital wants the patient out! The patient and family may not feel ready to leave, or they may disapprove of the proposed arrangements. Sometimes the attending physician will intervene to extend the hospital stay, but his power is limited because medical decisions of that nature are reviewed by the hospital's utilization committee. If there have been unusual medical circumstances or complications other days can be applied for through Medicare. These so called "outliers" can be approved for payment. The hospital can also apply for **administratively necessary days** if the patent cannot be placed before the scheduled discharge date.

The hospital, however, has weapons which it can direct at the patient. If the patient or his family objects to the discharge arrangements, the hospital can turn the patient's name into Medicare and ask for a listing of "uncooperative family." Medicare benefits can be terminated. In extreme instances, the hospital can apply to the courts for a **conservator of the person.** If they win, this new guardian can make arrangements for the patient.

Although hospital administrations may threaten to use their "big guns," it is doubtful that they will aggressively pursue challenging Medicare benefits or court actions. Few courts would take guardianship away from a concerned family except under exceptional circumstances.

RULE 5: OBTAIN A COMPLETE UNDERSTANDING OF THE PATIENT'S MEDICAL CONDITION AND PROGNOSIS

Once the question of alternative living arrangements has been raised, a conference should be held with the patient's doctor. It is imperative that you obtain a clear understanding of the individual's medical problems and prognosis. Other health care workers may be involved in the care of the patient, but the physician is in the best position to draw it all together. Some of the questions to be asked are:

1. What are the patient's medical problems?
2. What are the names of each diagnosis in medical terms?
3. Can you explain each diagnosis in lay terms?
4. What drugs have you prescribed?
   What is the purpose of each?
   What are the side effects?
5. What physical limitations does the patient have?
6. What mental limitations does the patient have?
7. Is there any evidence of confusion?
8. Are nursing services required, and if so, for how many hours a day?
9. Are there any special devices available that would enhance the patient's mobility and independence at home?
10. What future predictions can be made about the patient's medical course?
11. Is a consultation with a specialist indicated? (e.g., a consult with a urologist for incontinence.)
12. Is a visit to a geriatric assessment center necessary or available to the patient?

If the physician is unable to answer certain questions he should make appropriate referrals. Some elderly people will be receiving care from several specialists and therapists, all of whom may have a different perspective on the patient. Thus, maintaining a close relationship with the primary care physician is important.

GERIATRIC ASSESSMENT CENTERS
GERIATRIC ASSESSMENT UNITS, GERIATRIC EVALUATION CLINICS

Some of the larger metropolitan hospitals, particularly teaching hospitals associated with medical schools, have established geriatric assessment centers. These interdisciplinary units perform a complete physical and psychological evaluation on the individual. In order to locate such a center, contact your physician or telephone the nearest large medical center and ask for their department of geriatrics or gerontology.

After an application is made to an assessment unit, social workers and nurses will contact the patient and pertinent family members for basic information. A request will also be made to the physician for a copy of the medical records. A case manager, usually a social worker, is then assigned.

A medical workup is performed by gerontologists and other specialists. Interviews are arranged with social workers familiar with health care facilities. If needed, occupational, physical and speech therapists will be asked to see the patient in consultation. Neuropsychologic testing is common and can often clarify the presence and magnitude of dementia.

The case manager, utilizing information obtained from the physicians, therapists and tests, meets with the family and patient to discuss the group's recommendations. A copy of this summary is also sent to the patient's primary care physician. In some instances, the conclusion of the assessment may be that nursing home placement is indicated.

PRIVATE GERIATRIC CASE MANAGERS

A newly discovered, yet rapidly growing niche, has been filled by private geriatric case managers. They perform a useful function particularly if there is geographic distance between elderly parents and their children. The manager will locate and coordinate social services, arrange home care if necessary and even select and arrange admission to a nursing home. Their role is similar to the case manager in a geriatric assessment unit, except that their relationship is long–term and of a broader scope.

Their fees, which **are** *not* covered by Medicare or private insurance policies, range from $40 to $120 per hour, and some charge an initial assessment fee of $100 to $500.

Because of the newness of this field, there are no regulations or established criteria for qualifications or certification. It is suggested that you check their references and background carefully and obtain a written contract of services to be rendered along with cost estimates.

The recently formed National Association of Private Geriatric Case Managers (NAPGCM) has nearly 300 full members located in 47 states. Full members of this organization are individuals who devote full time to the field. They are prepared to offer assessment, counseling, crisis intervention, placement, advocacy, case management, entitlements consultation, information and referral and other services.

A list of members in your area can be obtained by writing or calling NAPGCM, 1315 Talbut Tower, Dayton, Ohio, 45402. 513-222-2621.

RULE 6: ASSESS MEDICAL CARE NEEDS AGAINST AVAILABLE RESOURCES

After a conference with the primary care physician and others, a list of health care needs can be developed. Family resources and available community agencies can be tallied and compared against needs.

When resources exceed needs, home care and independent living, assuming this is a safe option, are feasible. Homemaking chores must also be considered. These can range from simple tasks, such as a weekly grocery shopping trip or twice daily dog walking, to complex requirements—the need for a full–time homemaker or health aide. To obtain a professional opinion about home health care, **contact a home health care agency** and arrange for their free appraisal. There is excellent literature available on how to select a home health care agency, or you can simply choose one that is Medicare approved. The local **visiting nurse service** can also offer advice on the level of home care required.

Any consideration of home care is not appropriate if there is no convenient home in which to provide the care. If the elderly individual cannot safely live without constant supervision or is manifesting signs which indicate independent living is becoming too difficult, home care is not an option.

If need exceeds resources, then placement in a nursing home is required. A custodial care facility would be sufficient for those individuals who have few nursing needs yet require a safe environment, and for others who need minor assistance for some of the activities of daily living. The level of nursing care required determines whether a skilled nursing home placement is needed. Most physicians should be able to help a family decide what type of nursing home is needed.

RULE 7: EXPLORE YOUR FEELINGS ABOUT THE PLACEMENT
Ruth L., 78

Ruth lived an independent life in her apartment only a few blocks away from her daughter. Her mind was clear, although she suffered from Parkinson's disease. Because of the Parkinson's she had a resting tremor in her hands, walked with a stooped, shuffling gait and took a while to communicate her thoughts. Her daughter, a high school teacher, visited three times each week after school was over. During these visits, they went grocery shopping together, kept doctor's appointments and ran other errands.

Recently the family physician told her daughter, Marge, that Ruth's body was covered with bruises, most likely from several falls. The doctor feared that the next fall might lead to a fractured hip. When questioned, Ruth admitted to Marge that she had been falling, usually at night when she went to the bathroom. The falls were increasing, but she vowed to be more careful in the future.

That night Marge called her brother, Arnold, a hard–driving businessman who lived several thousand miles away in California, and informed him of their mother's condition. A few days later Arnold flew to his mother's city to verify the facts for himself. Both brother and sister agreed that their mother could not continue to live alone without supervision.

"There just isn't room in our house," Arnold told Marge over dinner. "Now that my girls are teenagers they each have their own room. Helen has a damn fine job with the real estate company, and I can't expect her to quit and baby–sit Mom."

"My condo just isn't large enough," Marge replied.

"Sell it and buy a larger one."

"The market is soft right now. It would be easier for you to build an addition on your house."

"Someone will still have to watch over her," Arnold said. He looked pensive a moment before continuing sheepishly. "The truth of the matter is, you know that Mom and Helen never got along. Helen told me before I left California that if I brought her home, she'd leave."

"I have a chance to be chairperson of my department next year," Marge said.

"You get along with her, and besides, you're a woman. You can do the necessary things."

"And you're still sexist!" Marge snapped. "What you mean is, home care is 'sister care,' Being female is not an automatic qualification for doing 'necessary things.' "

"Damn it!" Arnold exploded. "She gave birth to us. I'll be damned if I'll admit we can't take care of her now that she needs us."

"Maybe we should look around for a nursing home?" Marge suggested.

"My mother will never go to a home!" Arnold said.

"Then you had better start looking for a new wife," his sister said.

They were both silent for a few moments. "We're both a couple of SOBs, aren't we?" Arnold said softly.

Arnold and Marge are not as selfish as they think they are. They are faced with real and difficult problems. Although they are attempting to fit the care of their mother into one of the two home situations, neither is convenient or practical. Before this dilemma is resolved, Arnold will probably have a huge fight with his wife, and Marge will attempt to sell her condominium and buy a larger unit. They suffer from the pangs of guilt and will continue to do so until the crisis has been resolved.

The trauma of guilt can be further complicated if the elderly person involved wishes to play manipulative games. We overheard this gem from an older woman talking with her children:

"I will never live with strangers as long as you children can give me a crust of bread and a cup of cold coffee each day."

Some people have manipulated their family and friends throughout their lives. In those instances, you can merely recognize the game and insulate yourself as much as possible. Guilt trips are invoked by another distinct group of the elderly: those who already feel estranged and isolated from their family and desperately seek to hold on to what little remains.

Guilt exists in many forms and is the primary family emotion that affects the nursing home decision, visitation, the adjustment period and death. It evokes resentment which leads to anger and to more guilt—a self–perpetuating cycle. Only acknowledgment of its presence through introspection, family discussions and counseling, if necessary, will permit a family to overcome guilt's destructive effects.

There is a myth in our culture which states that if a family can take care of four toddlers they can certainly care for one elderly adult. This argument ignores the progression of children: The terrible twos eventually become the placid threes; children can be toilet trained; they learn to talk; and they usually sleep through the night.

The family dynamics of middle–aged children and their parents have evolved over decades, and spouses are not part of this interaction. A live–in elderly parent has the potential to tear a family apart. As the patient requires increasing amounts of attention, marital equilibrium may be put in jeopardy. The emotional survival of a family and marriage must be considered as carefully as an independent elderly person's safety: Neither should be sacrificed.

The families of prospective residents must explore their feelings about placement, realizing that a sense of guilt is usual, and that survival of the remaining family unit is also of prime importance.

RULE 8: REALIZE THAT GOOD NURSING HOMES DO EXIST

The nursing home industry has not just had bad press; it has received media coverage that makes turn of the century muck rakers seem like apologists for child labor and sweatshops. During the research of this book, we did not find a single article in the popular press which favorably portrayed nursing homes. Most journalists delight in pointing to the apparently ubiquitous abuse of the elderly.

There are nursing homes whose walls enclose dumping grounds for the aged. There are institutions where the treatment is so bad that the very will to live is drained. Fragile patients in these settings become more fragile, the continent become incontinent, the mobile turn immobile. Their residents suffer from pressure sores (a result of nursing inattention), and these facilities have intolerant help and inadequate nutrition.

Susan Sandel, a nursing home administrator in Connecticut, wrote the following in the *New York Times* on March 12, 1989:

> *To understand why America is so intent on the shaming of its elders one must look back at the history of the nursing home industry in this country. While hospitals grew out of medical science, nursing homes developed out of the welfare system. Long-term care institutions evolved from poor houses for the indigent and various charitable living arrangements provided by religious and secular groups.*
>
> *Americans traditionally have difficulty accepting and dealing with nonproductive segments of society. We typically identify problematic populations (orphans, the mentally ill and elderly), create institutions for their care and then*

denigrate those institutions for inhumane and inadequate care when they do
not meet public expectations.

The explosion in the numbers of nursing homes occurred with the passage of the Older American's Act in the mid–1960s. With the establishment of Medicare and especially Medicaid, which finances a tremendous number of nursing home beds, countless unscrupulous operators entered the field. At that time these facilities were barely regulated and many abuses, financial and personal, occurred. Investigative reporters had a field day, exposés abounded, people went to jail, and finally the regulators began to regulate.

Federal and state nursing home regulations are now monitored carefully by state agencies, usually under the auspices of the State Department of Health. Within the limitations of present day operating procedures and problems, ***poor skilled nursing homes are not the rule, but the exception***. The single most significant cause of poor care is a hardship endured by the industry as a whole: inadequate and poorly trained personnel. It is the task of the prospective resident's advocate to avoid the poor establishments and select the adequate or superior facility.

RULE 9: PROVIDE SUPPORT TO A PERSON ENTERING A NURSING HOME

Most significant passages in life have formal tribal rites that enable individuals to gather the support of their family friends and community. Examples include childbirth, baptism, bar mitzvahs, graduations, weddings, anniversaries, retirements and funerals. Entrance into a nursing home is an awkward transition made without appropriate ceremony. People do not feel good about the decision, and residents may feel abandoned and isolated. Our culture has not developed the ritual to deal with this type of passage.

Support can be provided in many ways. Making the decision a mutual one forms the basis for a supportive relationship. Spending as much time as possible with the prospective residents actively reassures them that their family has not abandoned them. Including all family members in the decision while maintaining a primary spokesperson presents an undivided front. Openly discussing everyone's feelings about the placement enhances understanding of each other's situation.

RULE 10: UNDERSTAND THAT THE NURSING HOME PLACEMENT CAN BE A GOOD DECISION

Because we have a horrid perception of the "home" and our culture has not adequately dealt with the period between retirement and death, it is hard to view the decision of placement as good. We assume that our friends will think in the same vein. "What will they think if we put Mom in one of those places?'' This is a question often asked either openly or subconsciously. Our friends are probably more tolerant and understanding than we expect. In all probability they are asking themselves the same type of question.

Good nursing homes can be found. Because of the increased number and changing complexion of the health of the elderly, more chronic diseases and older individuals, long-term care facilities are necessary. Modern families are not equipped for years of caring for an infirm elder. Even so, placement into a nursing home does not equal abandonment. Frequent visitation is important for nursing home residents to overcome their tendency to feel isolated.

Nursing homes ensure the safety of the patient and deliver the appropriate medical and nursing care. Many residents, once acclimated to their new surroundings, become more social and develop new friendships with staff and other residents.

CHAPTER 3

WHAT'S IN A NAME?

SOME BASIC DEFINITIONS

WHERE ARE THE
NURSING HOMES?

A rose is a rose is a rose, and it may be the same flower by other names, but try to find a nursing home without knowing where to look! The term is confusing, so do the obvious and turn to the yellow pages of any telephone directory.

A typical yellow page listing under "nursing homes" refers the searcher to the "convalescent home" listing. Under that listing we might find a group such as:

Aaron Manor Health Care Facility
Beechwood Manor, Inc.
Chestelm
Chesterfields Chronic and Convalescent Hospital
Deep River Convalescent Home.
Harbor Crossing Skilled Nursing Care Facility
Pettipaug Manor
Watrous Nursing Center, Inc.

The listings above are a mixture of various types of facilities which deliver different levels of care and provide services for diverse types of patients. It is difficult to tell by a name exactly what level of nursing skill is delivered. The situation becomes even more confused when other terms are put forth, such as acute care facility, skilled nursing home, chronic care hospital, life care facility, long–term care institution, extended care, rest home, intermediate care facility, homes for the aged and custodial care facilities.

Many of these terms overlap, others are synonymous and a few do not have real meaning in today's health care delivery system.

ACUTE CARE FACILITY
THE GENERAL HOSPITAL

The acute care hospital can range in size from the 20–bed rural facility to a large metropolitan medical complex. Medical centers which are associated with medical and nursing schools are termed teaching hospitals. The general hospital is divided into several patient care services: medicine, surgery, psychiatry, pediatrics and obstetrics/gynecology. Each of these divisions admits patients to certain areas of the hospital called wards or units. Thus, there are medical wards, surgical wards, etc. The epicenter of the ward is the nurse's station. This is where the patient's records are kept, doctors communicate with each other and where nursing reports occur.

People are admitted to an acute care hospital because of a sudden onset of illness or a rapid deterioration of a chronic disease. Critically ill patients are placed in an intensive care unit, while others are admitted to the appropriate wards. The medical care rendered is much more intensive than that received at a nursing home. Vital signs are taken frequently, physicians make daily rounds, and the wards are filled with licensed nurses. The activity level is very high and often harried. Elderly people, especially those who are confused, can easily be overwhelmed by this milieu. Yet, some family members prefer it to a nursing home for the patient will receive a great deal of attention. They should realize that hospitals specialize in treating physical illness, and should be utilized as little as possible in the care of the elderly.

REHABILITATION CENTERS

Facilities for rehabilitation centers are often a part of a large medical center or associated with such a complex. Admission is usually directly from the acute care hospital on the recommendation of the patient's attending physician and an evaluation by a team of specialists in rehabilitation medicine. The high goals of these centers which often require intense staff efforts and patient stamina do not always make them a viable alternative for the frail elderly.

Typical patients at a rehabilitation center are victims of strokes or traumatic accidents, and some facilities accept individuals who require mechanical ventilation. The patients must be cooperative, mentally alert and able to work with the specialists for several hours a day.

These centers, often through heroic effort, can upgrade the quality of life for their participants, but entrance into them is a medical determination and does not fall into the scope of this book.

Skilled nursing homes will have rehabilitative services available. Their goals may be slightly less auspicious, but remarkable strides can be made under the right circumstances.

TYPES OF NURSING HOMES

Until recently the federal government, through its Medicare and Medicaid regulations, recognized two types of nursing homes: *skilled* care facilities and *intermediate* care facilities. The major difference between the two was the amount and level of nursing care available to each patient. As a practical matter, patients in intermediate facilities were usually ambulatory and continent, and did not require extensive nursing treatments. The distinction between the two types of home was often quite arbitrary.

It had long been felt that this type of categorization was a false distinction, and as a matter of practicality, many institutions mixed both levels of care as multi–level facilities.

It is necessary for those investigating nursing homes to know of this past distinction because some advertising and other references to nursing homes will still carry these labels.

The federal government now refers to Medicare or Medicaid approved homes as skilled nursing facilities. The various state agencies involved in this field (Departments of Health, Welfare and Aging) will also refer to them as skilled nursing homes and/or chronic or convalescent homes.

Some states also recognize and license a second category of nursing home (what in the past was the third category) which are called by various names, such as rest homes, homes for the aged, custodial care institutions, residential adult care centers or board and care centers. These are not a federally recognized category of nursing home, and many states do not regulate them. In some instances, the only control over them is through local health officers—which means virtually no control at all.

SKILLED NURSING HOMES
CHRONIC AND CONVALESCENT CARE

The individual states are in charge of enforcing federal regulations concerning Medicare and Medicaid approved nursing homes. Many states adopt the federal standards as their own, while other states have more stringent requirements.

The keystone of these regulations is that a registered nurse be on duty during the day shift, and that licensed nurse coverage be available on a 24–hour basis. There are numerous other regulations concerning all aspects of the home's construction, fire safety, personnel definitions, etc., which will be considered in appropriate detail in chapters four and five.

Simply defined, the skilled nursing home is a health care facility with continuous licensed nurse coverage with the capabilities of providing around–the–clock nursing treatments as ordered by the patient's physician.

It must be noted that some nursing homes choose not to be Medicare and Medicaid approved; however, in most states the licensure requirements for all skilled nursing homes are identical, and care must be taken to establish this fact if a home under consideration is not Medicare approved.

CUSTODIAL HOMES
REST HOMES, HOMES FOR THE AGED, RESIDENTIAL ADULT CARE CENTERS, ADULT FOSTER CARE, BOARD AND CARE

Institutions known as custodial homes provide safe surroundings for the ambulatory elderly who are self–medicating, continent and alert. Residents must be able to self–transfer and walk at least a few steps without aid, but may use assistive devices such as canes, walkers and wheelchairs.

Custodial homes provide full meal service and recreational activities. This type of alternative living arrangement is for the non–frail elderly who do not or cannot live at home, but who are not chronically incapacitated. It is a more protected environment than elderly or congregate housing, and allows the residents to live without concern over homemaker services.

THE HOSPICE

Palliative and supportive care for terminally ill patients is provided by the hospice. The emphasis is on controlling pain, and dealing with the emotional and spiritual problems of death and dying. These organizations are considered in depth in chapter 13.

THE NURSES

In the nursing home setting, as in any other hospital setting, the nursing staff delivers the majority of health services. It is the nurses and aides who care for the patient on a day–to–day, hour–by–hour schedule. These are the individuals that can greatly influence the patient's health and quality of life.

But who are they?

REGISTERED NURSE (RN)

There are three ways to receive the education necessary for taking the registered nurse licensing examination:

1. A bachelor of science degree in nursing from an approved four year college.
2. A certificate of nursing received from an approved nursing school affiliated with a general hospital. These courses are usually three years in length and have about the same number of hours of science courses and clinical work as the BSN, but not the other undergraduate courses the usual college graduate would normally take.
3. A two year certificate in nursing. Graduates of these short courses have little clinical experience. They are sometimes hired by health care facilities on an internship basis until they have more clinical exposure. Graduates of these programs often have difficulty with their licensing examinations because of their lack of clinical experience.

A general duty nurse is an RN without specialized training. Many nurses continue their education in graduate programs or take specialized training in such fields as pediatrics, surgical nursing, gerontology, public health or other fields.

LICENSED PRACTICAL NURSE (LPN)
ALSO KNOWN AS LICENSED VOCATIONAL NURSE (LVN) IN TEXAS AND CALIFORNIA)

A licensed practical nurse has attended a practical nursing program for a year or a year and a half, and then passed a national proficiency examination. LPN courses stress a clinical approach, and most LPNs have the same clinical experience as an RN, but they do not have the science background of the RN. LPNs work under the supervision of RNs, and in nursing homes they are capable of performing all treatments, administering medications and performing the majority of other nursing functions.

Because of the acute shortage of RNs throughout the country, and the type of nursing treatments required, the majority of nurses encountered in a nursing home will be LPNs. Federal regulations require RN supervision during the day shift, but LPN or RN coverage for the remaining hours.

NURSE'S AIDES
NURSING ASSISTANTS

The people who provide the hour by hour care to nursing home patients are called nurse's aides. They help feed, bathe, change and dress patients. An aide cannot give medications or perform nursing treatments.

Present federal regulations now require that aides be certified. Previously, nursing homes provided 75-hour in-house training programs toward that certification. Now, certification is often obtained through technical schools, junior colleges, and other educational organizations.

DIRECTOR OF NURSING

The director of nursing is in charge of all nursing personnel and aides, and is responsible for coordinating all nursing programs and implementing patient care plans. She is in charge of scheduling, discipline and hiring of nursing personnel. In large institutions she will often have one or more assistants.

CHARGE NURSE

Each nursing unit, usually consisting of 30 patients, will have a charge nurse on duty at all times. This nurse is responsible for seeing that all assignments are kept, and that medications are properly delivered. In addition to supervising the nursing assistants, the charge nurse is responsible for patient charting and overseeing that all physician's orders are carried out.

THERAPISTS

There is an army of support personnel to aid the nursing home patients. The availability of these services is mandated by Medicare and Medicaid regulations, but depending on the size of the facility, they may be delivered by part–time personnel. Therapists are highly skilled rehabilitation specialists who have received years of training in their fields. Also working in the various disciplines are assistant level personnel who handle the more routine cases.

PHYSICAL THERAPISTS (PT)

Rehabilitation specialists known as physical therapists work with patients to help them regain or retain maximal use of specific muscle groups. They may devise regimens which focus on improving the range of motion of a joint in a patient with arthritis, re–establishing a gait in a stroke victim or continuing activity while an immobilized patient remains in bed. Physical therapists are particularly adept at personalizing ambulation equipment: canes, crutches, walkers and if needed, wheelchairs. Each nursing home should have a physical therapy room with essential equipment: whirlpool tubs, an ambulation training area with mats, parallel bars and possibly an equipment workshop.

OCCUPATIONAL THERAPISTS (OT)

The occupational therapist teaches patients how to adapt themselves to perform activities of daily living—in other words, daily occupations. They adjust the skills they teach depending on the patient's condition. OTs also ingeniously construct novel devices that assist patients with activities of daily living. For example, a patient who has suffered a stroke may have profound weakness on one side, but strength and coordination will gradually return to the affected limbs. During the initial phase of recovery, the OT may train the patient to use a buttoning device which requires use of a single hand. As function returns to the affected hand, the assist device may be discarded and buttoning tricks will be taught, so that the affected hand is used as much as possible.

It is apparent that the functions of the PT and OT should merge. A recovering stroke patient, as an example, should work closely with both therapists to recover all possible functions.

Speech Therapist (ST)

Anyone who has difficulty chewing or swallowing food or with speech will require the services of a speech therapist. They commonly work with stroke victims who are aphasic or have swallowing dysfunction. STs are skilled in developing and teaching the use of alternative communication devices. Aphasic patients may be unable to articulate words, but they may be competent in the use of a speech board (a device containing letters so that words can be spelled by pointing). STs are also well versed on the types of food to give a patient with a recovering swallowing function.

Recreational Therapist
Therapeutic Recreation Specialist, Patient Activities Coordinator

Medicare and Medicaid approved homes must have a qualified recreational director on staff and publish a calendar of scheduled events. These activities should vary and have a broad interest range in order to provide meaningful activity for patients at all levels of physical and mental ability.

Podiatrist (DPM)
Doctor of Podiatric Medicine

A college graduate who has four years of additional training at a recognized school of podiatry is a podiatrist. An important member of the medical team for the elderly, he can medicate and perform treatments or surgery on the foot, usually up to the ankle.

Dietician
Nutritionist, Registered Dietician (RDs)

The nutritionist will assess a patient's dietary needs, evaluate current diets and plan a nutritional program to promote the health of the patient within the guidelines of medical needs. In some instances the dietician will prepare diets to conform to religious requirements. The type of diet, such as NAS (no added salt), ADA (American Diabetic Association), soft, clear, liquid or mechanical, will be ordered by the physician.

FOOD SERVICE MANAGER
(IN A SMALL NURSING HOME, THE COOK.)

The food service manager is in charge of food purchase and supervision of kitchen personnel, and has responsibility for all food preparation as scheduled by the dietician.

SOCIAL WORKER (MSW)

Most nursing homes will have a full– or part–time social worker who will know how to tap into community services and give aid in case management. The social worker can give advice on Medicare and Medicaid, and also act as a patient advocate in other areas. The social worker should be able to counsel and support families during emotionally difficult times.

NURSING HOME ADMINISTRATOR

The administrator is the senior supervisor of the nursing home, and will usually have done graduate work in the health care field. He or she will often be a member of the professional organization, The American College of Health Care Administrators. The administrator is licensed by the state and is the individual ultimately responsible for all that happens within the institution. As a practical matter, the administrator's primary duties tend to be in the areas of personnel management, fiscal planning and purchasing. In larger nursing homes there might be one or more assistant administrators, each having specific areas of responsibility.

THE DOCTORS

Those of us who grew up with fictional Doctors, know that physicians go to college where they study pre–medical sciences, attend medical school and then intern for a year before going forth into the world to do good things.

Modern medical education, like the rest of medicine, has changed. Today's potential doctors major in biology, chemistry, history or any number of academic disciplines while undergraduates. Admission to medical school requires a core group of courses in biology, chemistry, physics and mathematics. The first two years of medical school are academic in nature and consist of lectures and laboratory science. The final two years of medical school utilize hospital–based clinical rotations as the major teaching tool.

Groups of medical students often congregate around patients' beds while being taught by a senior physician, who extracts answers by using the Socratic method of teaching. Medical students may be called student doctors, young physicians, physicians, physicians in training or externs (fourth–year students who function as interns).

After graduation from medical school, the new doctor spends at least three years in a residency program, although certain specialties can require as many as five years of post–graduate training. These residencies are in the familiar specialties of internal medicine, pediatrics, radiology, family practice and others. After completion of their residency, many physicians elect to specialize further and continue as "fellows." An example of this further specialization would be an internist accepting a two year fellowship in geriatrics. Therefore, a geriontologist has completed four years of college, four years of medical school, three years of an internal medicine residency and two years of a fellowship, a total of 13 years of training.

ATTENDING PHYSICIAN

The attending physician is the patient's doctor of record, however, he or she may or may not be your doctor of choice in a nursing home situation. If the patient's personal physician has admitting privileges at the selected nursing home, then he or she can continue as attending physician. If your doctor is not on the home's list, the nursing home administrators will ask that you select another physician from those allowed to attend at that institution. The fact that doctors do not have privileges at a given institution is not necessarily a reflection on competency. It may mean that this is the first time a patient of theirs has been admitted to that institution, or that the nursing home is inconveniently located. It may also mean that the owner or administrator of the nursing home has chosen to limit the number of doctors providing care. It would obviously be inconvenient to have an unlimited number of attending physicians, but it is also true that utilizing a short list from which choices are made can be beneficial for those on that list. The home's medical director, who is also a doctor in private practice, is often the physician who is selected by unaffiliated patients.

Attending physicians are medically responsible for patients. They must write all medical orders. A do–not–resuscitate order can only be written by the attending physician. Any important medical decision is ultimately made by this physician in consultation with the patient and family.

OUR DOCTOR ISN'T GIVING US ENOUGH INFORMATION OR—WHY DOCTORS DON'T HELP MORE IN THE NURSING HOME DECISION

Your doctor is probably a member of a group practice or an HMO (Health Maintenance Organization). Such a participant is a member of a team effort.

A group might include any number of doctors, and each of its internists will often have their own specialty. As the elderly begin to develop certain infirmities such as arthritis, heart problems or any number of complaints, they might be referred from one member of the group to another for treatment of that particular problem. Although this system is more efficient in many ways and does allow for a more educated delivery of health care services, it also reduces the amount of time a patient spends with any one doctor. As a consequence the personal relationship between doctor and patient suffers, and the individual physician does not see the whole person.

Holistic medicine is becoming a thing of the past. Our relationship with our physician is far more formal, and without knowledge of our family, finances and personality, the doctor is far more reluctant to deliver authoritative pronouncements.

Even the sole practitioner in family practice medicine is apt to make referrals for certain medical problems. The rise of malpractice litigation has virtually dictated this procedure.

In addition to the loss of doctor–patient relationships, another factor must be considered: Many doctors just don't like geriatric medicine. It seems ironic that with the rise in our elderly population that our medical profession shows decreasing interest in their physical problems. There are several reasons for this attitude:

1. The elderly are apt to suffer from more than one chronic complaint and the time required for individual attention is longer than for younger patients.
2. Payment by the elderly is apt to be Medicare or Medicaid which is less than can be charged for similar services to self–pay or privately insured patients.
3. HMO organizations which are funded by set monthly fees are interested in preventative medicine as this increases their profit. HMOs with large numbers of elderly patients are far less profitable.
4. The elderly do not respond dramatically to the miracles of modern medicine. Doctors like to cure people. They know that practice with the elderly is a holding pattern at best, and slow or rapid deterioration at worst. The very nature of medical training tends to steer the most idealistic physicians away from geriatric medicine.
5. Paradoxical as it may seem, considering the demographics of the elderly, geriatrics has only recently become a recognized specialty. It is true that teaching hospitals have offered fellowships for several years, but it was not until 1988 that a certifying examination signifying competence in geriatric medicine was given. It is astonishing to realize that the first department of geriatrics in an American medical school was not established until Mount Sinai in New York City began its program in 1982.

MEDICAL DIRECTOR

The medical director is a physician charged with the responsibility for the assurance of quality medical care in the facility, and to act as liaison between the medical staff and the administration. He must make sure that each patient has a physician, and provide or arrange care if the patient's individual doctor is unable or unwilling to do so. He receives reports from the director of nurses on significant clinical developments.

NURSING HOME OWNERSHIP

Since 1974 there has been a 38% increase in nursing home beds, but even with this expansion, these facilities are averaging a 92% occupancy rate on a national basis. The 1,624,200 beds are divided amongst some 25,000 different categories of nursing homes which are owned as outlined in Figure 4.

Beverly Enterprises, Inc., is the largest nursing home chain in the country and once owned 1,003 homes containing 109,000 beds. Due to financial difficulties, in 1989 they sold 370 homes containing 38,000 beds. Other major nursing home chains are Manor Care with 20,000 beds, and National Medical Enterprises with 43,000 beds. Smaller corporations might own only a few facilities while many are held in small corporations comprising one nursing home.

Non-profit or voluntary homes are those owned by religious, fraternal or charitable groups chartered under appropriate state laws. By definition they cannot return or distribute profits to any individual or corporation. These homes, because they offer residents a homogeneous group, have an immediate sense of community to the resident or family. Since they are backed financially by the parent organization, their care is often excellent, but paradoxically their rates are usually higher than the profit-making homes. Nonetheless, they tend to have the longest waiting lists.

Federal and state owned homes include nursing home beds reserved in Veteran's Administration hospitals, state "Old Soldier's Homes," the last vestiges of "county homes," and other small mixes of publicly funded facilities.

Geographically these nursing homes are located as shown in Figure 5.

It is important to note that Figures 4 and 5 do not include numerous custodial or board and care facilities that are not supervised by federal regulations, and in many instances are not under state supervision.

FIG. 4: NURSING HOME OWNERSHIP

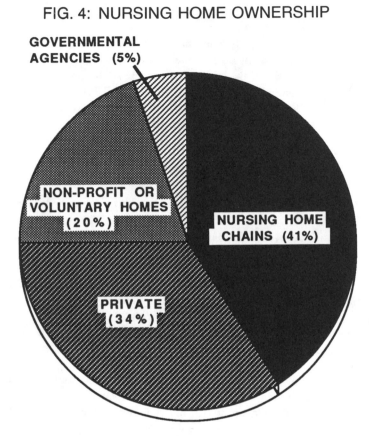

Source: National Nursing Home Survey, 1985

HEALTH MAINTENANCE ORGANIZATIONS (HMO)

HMOs are a method of prepaying health service costs, which usually include physician's charges, prescription drugs and lab tests. For a monthly fee paid to the group, an individual is entitled to these services without further charge or with a minor copayment fee.

There are two basic types of HMOs:

Closed: in which case the physicians work exclusively for that particular HMO, and often the labs and pharmacy will be a part of the organization.

Open: doctors under contract to the HMO provide medical services to the

FIG. 5: GEOGRAPHIC DISTRIBUTION OF NURSING HOMES IN THE UNITED STATES

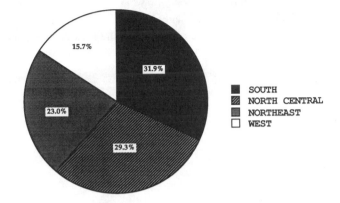

■ SOUTH
▨ NORTH CENTRAL
▤ NORTHEAST
☐ WEST

Source: National Nursing Home Survey, 1985

members, but also provide care to other patients on a fee–for–service basis. Lab tests and drugs are provided to the HMO by an approved group of providers.

The growth of these organizations has been explosive. Numbering barely 13 in 1964, there were 607 by the 1980s, and since 1983 their membership has tripled until they now serve over 32.5 million patients. This rapid growth has not been without problems. Many HMOs, to meet competitive factors, lowered rates, underwrote groups that were not economically viable and consequently suffered severe financial hardships and bankruptcies.

Whether the HMO is open or closed, individuals are usually able to select their own primary physicians, providing those doctors are members of the group.

The growth of these organizations has been due to several factors:

1. Large corporations that provide health benefits for their employees found that they were riding a spiral of increasing costs. HMOs seemed to answer that problem by practicing preventative medicine and by not ordering unneeded tests. Also, HMOs were more responsive to large companies' needs because of the number of members they could deliver.
2. Operating in an open or closed HMO, doctors' billing and collection problems were simplified, and their patient numbers were guaranteed.

Numerous studies seem to indicate that HMOs provide as good if not better health care delivery than the traditional pay–as–you–go models. The problems with these groups, once again, has been economic, not medical, mismanagement.

Medicare refers to these groups as "prepayment plans," and many of them have arrangements with Medicare. Home care under these circumstances would have to be along established Medicare guidelines.

CHAPTER 4

HOW TO CHOOSE

SELECTING A NURSING HOME

THE LEVEL OF CARE

The sections of this book dealing with selecting a nursing home are primarily directed toward the skilled facility. The most stringent requirements must be utilized for that level of care. It is in that situation where the patient is most apt to suffer from one or more chronic disabilities, have the frailest nature and be the most vulnerable to the vagaries of staff and physical setting. The general criteria utilized are applicable for all levels of care, with the exception of diminished nursing staff for custodial type residents, and less emphasis on rehabilitation features when they are not needed.

If there is any question concerning the level of care necessary for any individual patient, the family physician can readily give advice on this matter. However, it must be kept in mind that larger nursing homes often have various levels of care housed in the same facility. It is therefore incumbent on the individual making the search to anticipate future care needs when evaluating any given nursing home. It is not uncommon for a resident to move from one floor to another, one care level to another, within the same home. It is also not uncommon for an institution that may provide glorious custodial care with magnificent recreational programs to have staffing deficiencies in their nursing department that make their skilled units untenable.

WHEN A HOUSE IS NOT A HOME
A CASE HISTORY OF A NURSING
HOME SEARCH

The Dahlstroms had been through the agonized process of making the nursing home decision. They were now convinced that Barbara's mother, Helga, would have her health needs best served in a nursing home. They had spoken with their doctor, a social worker in their town and an assistant minister of their church who specialized in matters of the elderly. They had been referred to several nursing homes. Initial telephone calls had reduced their list to two potential facilities that were within easy visiting distance and fell within their price range. They made both appointments for the same day and began their journey.

They were impressed by their initial view of the Riverside Convalescent Home. A long winding entrance drive swept up a gently sloped hill to a cul–de–sac near the front portico. The grounds were immaculate and well manicured, and arcs of water from recessed sprinklers attested to the lawn's continuing maintenance.

They were met in a chandeliered lobby by Donna, a bubbly, attractive woman in her mid–30s who represented the administrator's staff. Donna was their tour guide and was knowledgeable about the nursing home's facilities and the care they could offer Helga Dahlstrom, and seemed willing and able to answer all their questions.

They were pleased at the home's muted and placid atmosphere. The waxed and highly buffed floor reflected their image as they walked. The common rooms were spotless, well furnished and tastefully decorated like the lobby of a good hotel. The recreational, occupational and physical therapy rooms and card room held shelves of neatly stacked games, equipment and other necessary items.

Linen table cloths covered tables for four in the dining room, and the place settings were sterling with fluted goblets. The week's menu was posted near the dining room entrance and it revealed well balanced meals of an interesting variety.

The patients' semi–private rooms showed a decorator's touch. They were informed that depending on availability, there was a choice of three color schemes for the room, but most families were satisfied with any of the three.

A slight antiseptic smell permeated the building, but they were used to this from their knowledge of hospitals. They were favorably impressed, and knew they would feel no shame in having visitors see Helga Dahlstrom in this setting. Only reluctantly did they continue their search and drive to their next appointment at the Murphysville Chronic Convalescent Hospital.

THE HOUSE BUILT BY MAD ELVES

The Dahlstroms were shocked as they approached their next appointment.

The nursing home's attached buildings seemed to have been designed by mad elves. The much modified main structure appeared to have once been a Victorian mansion. Single story wings had been added over the years in starfish fashion. A chain link fence, topped with floodlights, fenced in the rear of the property and gave that portion of the property the look of a minimum security prison.

Reluctantly they entered the main building's reception area. A phalanx of wheelchairs filled with elderly patients was near the entrance; their occupants stared at them in open curiosity. There was a faint odor of recent urine in the air.

After an uncomfortable wait before the small army of wheelchairs and staring patients, they were finally taken in tow by a harried administrator. He steered them down patient–filled halls and negotiated them past groups in geri–chairs. Other residents made a slow progress toward some distant but unknown destination with walkers and canes. Nurses and aides bustled past, stopping occasionally to have a word with a patient.

A lone patient was still eating in the cluttered dining room. She ate with the fingers of one hand from a heavy plate which looked like a refugee from a roadside diner rather than a gourmet restaurant. In a corner of the dining room two elderly men and one woman energetically argued over the rules of a canasta game.

The patient's rooms, although of the same dimensions as those at Riverside, were a hodgepodge of pictures, odd pieces of furniture and stacks of personal belongings. If there had ever been any color coordination, it was submerged under the resident's possessions.

The Murphysville home was noisy and seemingly chaotic. The Dahlstroms were horrified and cut their visit as short as minimal social graces would allow.

Since the costs of both homes were similar, their choice was obvious. They would never allow Mother Dahlstrom to enter that "zoo" as they called the latter home. They would sign the contract with Riverside that very afternoon. They were pleased at their inspection tour, impressed with the good and the bad they had seen at each home, and told themselves that they had done well.

THE WRONG CHOICE

Well manicured lawns, spotless halls and showplace physical plants do not make a good nursing home. The Dahlstroms should have wondered how often the Riverside residents enjoyed those green lawns as they dodged the spray sprinklers hopscotching across the grass. It might also be possible that the pervasive antiseptic smell they noticed in home number one might have been utilized to cover lingering odors.

They should have been concerned at the quiet ambience of the first home and disturbed over the empty halls and common areas. The important questions they should have asked were:

Why were the residents not being ambulated?

Why were the residents not allowed in common areas?

Were the residents oversedated, which would account for the quiet aura in the home?

The neat stacks of occupational and recreational equipment might have meant an obsessive housekeeping staff, or it might have meant that the equipment was primarily for show rather than use.

The Riverside dining room was evidently a joy to behold, but did the actual meals served correspond to the posted menu? Fluted glasses and fine table settings are attractive, but are they practical for those recovering from strokes, those with tremors or others of the frail elderly who have difficulty with muscle coordination?

The second nursing home, haphazard as its exterior construction might appear, had a vitality about it which would make it more conducive to a congenial atmosphere. The unsightly rear yard was useful for confused patients who wished to spend time out–of–doors, but who might have wandered away without its fence.

This was obviously an active nursing home. Patients filled the halls and common areas, argued over card games and evidently were living lives as active as their medical conditions allowed. It was apparent that they were not oversedated or restrained. Although their rooms were not color coordinated, the decor meant that residents had brought many of their personal belongings in order to make each room unique to its inhabitants' personality.

A nursing home is just that—a home. It is a place where the patient will live for a few weeks to several years. The aura in the home, its physical plant, safety and housekeeping, will establish one important secondary set of qualities. It is the personnel of the facility, who in effect becomes the patient's extended family, who establish the first and most important measurement of quality.

How Do You Tell the Good From the Bad?
(Or the Good from the Mediocre?)

Once the placement decision has been made, either by patients, their spouses or some other trusted individual, the search begins. Because funds might be limited, and proximity to family is important, cost and geography are usually the initial considerations in choosing a nursing home.

If funds are limited, one might begin the initial search with those facilities listed as nonprofit organizations. However, it is usually incorrect to assume these homes will save you funds, as on a national average, nonprofit homes are more expensive than the profit making nursing facilities.

A nursing home with a specialized unit might be more important than geographic considerations. For example, a good nursing home with a separate Alzheimer's unit might prove more advantageous for the patient with that affliction than convenience for family visits.

Since cost and several medical conditions will be considered in depth in later chapters, let us assume that you have a choice of several facilities in your area. What are the first things you should look for?

THE FIRST SIX STEPS IN CHOOSING A NURSING HOME

STEP ONE: START YOUR LIST WITH MEDICARE–MEDICAID APPROVED NURSING HOMES

If at all possible, it is also recommended that the nursing home also be approved by the Joint Commission of Accreditation of Hospitals (JCAH). This approval is considered a definite plus, but is not an absolute necessity since many good nursing homes do not file for this accreditation. JCAH approval requires a thorough and independent inspection of the facility, the cost of which is paid by the nursing home. Since most nursing home owners consider themselves overregulated at best, and have no desire to spend additional funds for more regulation, many homes do not request this approval. Since many of the better homes are not JCAH approved, this standard can only be considered an additional protection if it is present, but not a deficiency if it is not.

If a nursing home is Medicare–Medicaid approved, it must adhere to certain minimal standards as set forth in the Federal Register. Since Medicaid is a joint venture between state and federal governments, each state has adopted minimal nursing home standards which are at least equal to the federal standards, but in several states are much more stringent than the national standards. The responsibility for inspecting and enforcing adherence to these regulations is almost always relegated to specialized nursing home inspection teams within the State Department of Health. These teams are primarily composed of registered nurses. They make periodic and unannounced visits to each nursing home in the state and follow–up inspections to see if deficiencies are corrected.

Although Medicare payments for long–term nursing home care are a small portion of the total fees. Medicaid, the joint federal–state entitlement program, pays a significant portion of the remaining costs. A nursing home stay can stretch into years, and except for the most affluent, the possibility of utilizing Medicaid at some future point must be anticipated. It is not uncommon for these lengthy stays to convert to Medicaid after depletion of the patient's available funds.

These are nursing homes which for financial reasons do not wish to be Medicare–Medicaid approved. However, creating an initial list with this approval as a criteria, not only provides future financial protection, but sets minimum standards as your starting point. A breakdown of the nation's 25,000 nursing homes indicates that 15,600 are medicare/medicaid approved.

Title 42—Public Health, of the Federal Register—is the published guideline for the establishment of skilled nursing homes. Section 405.1134 of that title concerns "Condition of Participation—Physical Environment." Among other things, this section establishes rules for fire protection, the necessity for emergency power and standard nursing units with call bells, and sets minimum requirements for patient rooms and toilet facilities. It also contains sections on dining and patient activity rooms, and the maintenance of grounds and equipment.

A glance at the patient room requirements reveals that they must be designed for patient care and privacy. They can have no more than four beds with a minimum of 80 square feet per bed. Each room is to be equipped with or located near adequate toilet and bathing facilities, and must have direct access to a corridor and outside exposure.

Although the federal standards allow four beds to a semi–private accommodation, it is recommended that two beds per room be the criteria of selection.

These regulations in their totality establish minimum standards in all phases of the nursing home operation from the qualifications necessary for a director of nursing to the establishment of proper disaster and evacuation plans. Focusing attention on homes operating under these standards means simply that one does not have to enter a nursing home with a clipboard filled with a thousand questions concerning the location of fire doors to the qualifications of the recreational director. The major items will be in place. Whether they are adequate and properly utilized is another question.

STEP TWO: LOOK AT THE STATE INSPECTION REPORTS

The nursing home administration is required to show interested people their last state inspection reports.

Request and digest these reports. Pay particular attention to nursing deficiencies rather than minor physical plant discrepancies. It is the job of nursing home inspectors to find fault, and they will. Many of the deficiencies cited will be minor, but continued lack of proper staffing, or an excessive rate of bedsores (decubiti) indicate major problems.

We know of one fine nursing home that was cited for having insufficient linen available. Staff members and patients knew that this was a temporary condition caused by the recent breakdown of the home's industrial washing machine. The condition was rectified on the following day after the machine's repair. Another good nursing home was cited for not posting a 911 emergency telephone number in the proper location. The inspector refused to acknowledge the fact that the locality did not have a 911 system at that time.

Mickey Mouse citations should be recognized for what they are, but serious and recurring violations should signal a poor home operating on the edge of disaster.

1988 National Survey of Nursing Home Deficiencies

Utilizing data compiled from reports prepared by the various state inspection teams, on December 1, 1988, the federal Department of Health and Human Services published a survey of the results. This 50 state, 75 volume report, investigated 32 performance area standards in over 15,000 nursing homes. This report was meant to act as a consumer's guide to nursing homes on a national basis.

The late Senator John Heinz of Pennsylvania, who was the ranking Republican member of the Select Committee on Aging, said, "Families in search of a quality nursing home may be frustrated if not out and out misguided by the data as presented in this report."

In order to place Senator Heinz's remarks in proper context as to the report, we considered one important citation. More than 4,000 of the 15,000 nursing homes investigated were found "to be administering drugs without regard to a physician's written order."

This deficiency would appear to have important concern. While we are not so naive as to believe that nursing homes in the United States represent the best of all possible alternative care for the elderly, it is also not possible to believe that 4,000 homes, nearly a quarter of the sample, blatantly dispensed drugs without a physician's order. Conferences with nursing home personnel and an investigation as to how this deficiency might have occurred raised the following possibilities:

1. Many, if not most, of the drug orders in the average nursing home setting are verbal orders taken over the telephone by the nurse from the physician. These orders are to be confirmed in writing in a timely manner, usually 48 hours. From a practical standpoint, often days will elapse between the order and the physician's signature in the chart.
2. Standing drug orders must be renewed every 30 days. The exigencies of the average physician's work day often preclude this renewal within the required time.
3. Certified nurse's aides in most states are allowed to administer SSEs (soap sud enemas), but not laxative suppositories. The administration of a suppository is considered a drug dispensing function.
4. A physician's order reads for tablets of Tylenol by mouth. The patient has a sore throat and the nurse administers an equivalent dose of liquid

Tylenol. Liquid instead of tablet would be a violation of the physician's orders.

5. Nurses without a physician's order administer a narcotic drug to a confused patient who is difficult to handle. This process, called snowing, is an absolute violation of all standards. But the report does not differentiate between this type of violation and the other four mentioned above.

Nursing home inspections serve a useful function. Eventually they will uncover the substandard nursing home and put its license in jeopardy. The inspection standards also set guidelines within the industry. They can also be misleading unless they are read in a manner that demonstrates patterns of violations that are detrimental to a patient's well–being.

STEP THREE: CHECK THE HOUSEKEEPING

Look at the nursing home as you would a hotel or motel room you were renting for a long anticipated vacation. The same standards which you would apply to your own housekeeping should be applicable, with two strong reservations:

Many of these patients never leave their rooms.
Two–thirds of the residents are partially or totally incontinent.

It is not unusual for there to be a smell of urine or feces in a nursing home. The important consideration is whether the odor is a stale smell of some duration or one of recent vintage. Nursing homes which have a strong smell of disinfectant or deodorizer might be using this to hide lingering odors. Time must also be considered. Testing the odors in a nursing home at 9:00 A.M. on a Monday morning is not a fair evaluation. At that hour the new shift (who arrived at 7:00) is in the midst of getting patients up for the day and completing breakfast. Clothing changes have to be made, bedding renewed and general housekeeping begun for the new week. Perhaps a batch of clean linen has not yet arrived on the unit since many institution launderies do not work weekends and Monday is catch–up day. It is recommended that a nursing home's odors be evaluated in the afternoon, by which time the flurry of morning activity should have abated.

STEP FOUR: CHECK ON THE FOOD

Anyone who has lived in any institutional setting, whether a college dorm, the army or a hospital, knows how important food is when other activities are constricted. Meal time is often the high point of the day, and this is certainly true in a nursing home.

Approved nursing homes are required to post their menus in a conspicuous location. It is important to check the meal actually served against the posted menu. The main meal of the day should be served at noon, with a lighter meal at night. Snacks, consisting of juice and perhaps a cookie should be available in the afternoon and at bedtime. The elderly can be overwhelmed by too much food. Their food intake and caloric needs are far less than for younger adults. The portions served should be adequate and balanced, but the large helpings provided in gourmet restaurants are not necessary.

The type of food served should be considered in relationship to the ability of the elderly to eat. A large steak might be enticing to a younger adult, while tender, easy to cut and chew pot roast would be more practical for the elderly with dentures or swallowing and chewing difficulties. The good nursing home will serve fresh fruits and vegetables when in season, and will not rely exclusively on prepared foods in their kitchen. The menu selection should be rotated on at least a three week cycle, although a four week cycle is recommended.

The food served should be varied, warm and attractively displayed, with an alternate main course. If possible, a meal should be sampled at the nursing home.

STEP FIVE: OBSERVE PATIENT ACTIVITY

One of the criticisms directed at nursing homes has been that they are our "warehouses for the elderly." Unfortunately, this stereotype can be true, yet it also is readily detected. This type of nursing home, similar to the one first described in this chapter's case history, will have the least patient activity. It is cheaper for the administration, and more convenient for the staff, if residents remain in their rooms and are not ambulated, dressed or moved. It is time consuming, and therefore more costly, to assist residents with transfers from bed to chair or wheelchair. It is far easier to perform the mundane tasks of self–care such as dressing or personal care for a patient, than it is to encourage him to do for himself. It is faster to feed a partially paralyzed patient than to aid him in the cumbersome task of relearning to feed himself. Life for the staff is easier if they can physically or chemically restrain a disruptive resident rather than allow him to roam the halls and common areas under supervision.

The poor nursing home will have far less resident activity than the better institution. In the good nursing home concerned with their residents' welfare, the patients will be up, and those who can will be in the halls or common areas utilizing canes, walkers or wheelchairs, if necessary. Unless it is medically impossible, each resident should be out of bed for long periods each day, as this enhances physical and emotional well–being.

STEP SIX: OBSERVE THE STAFF AND THEIR RELATIONSHIP TO THE RESIDENTS

The unit nurses and aides are the people with whom the resident lives on a day–by–day, hour–by–hour basis. They are the ones who provide the daily care, not the administrative staff or physicians.

Observation of the nursing staff's interaction with the residents will reveal more about the nursing home's qualifications than reading 50 inspection reports or eating a dozen meals in their dining room. The way the staff talks, touches and responds to patients will tell a great deal about how they will establish a relationship with the prospective resident. Rules cannot be created which will definitively bracket this nurse–patient relationship. Only a knowledge of human behavior will allow you to sense this feeling and determine whether it is of a positive or negative nature.

STAFF ADEQUACY

If the staff has a harried attitude and seems slightly impatient with the residents, and if patients are not ambulated or out of bed, the institution may be understaffed. Signs of poor or inadequate housekeeping, cold food and a high rate of bedsores are danger signals that point toward lack of adequate staff.

The greatest single problem facing the nursing home industry is the lack of adequate personnel. Nursing homes, like all other health care facilities, are faced with the dire shortage of registered nurses. Margretta Styles, president of the American Nurses Association, states that there is a shortage of 500,000 nurses. A recent survey by the American Health Care Association confirms that more than one in three nursing homes are grappling with a severe shortage of registered nurses. Twenty–three percent of nursing homes sampled report that they have a severe shortage of licensed practical nurses, while 56% rated the LPN shortage as moderate. Aide position vacancies are rated as severe in one of four homes, and moderate in 61% of the nursing homes.

Recent RN graduates tend to favor the acute care hospital for employment. They have a perception that this setting is more glamorous, and opt for further training in pediatrics, surgical nursing or other such specialties where medical results are often dramatic. LPNs, however, will often opt for geriatric nursing since their position in the medical hierarchy at a nursing home is higher than in an acute care hospital.

The attrition rate for nurses' aides and other nonlicensed personnel is often 100% a year. The task of transferring immobile patients is physically taxing, messy and poorly paid. A situation has been created where we have turned the care of our elderly over to underpaid, overworked aides who are compensated at the same hourly rate as a teenager at the nearest fast food chain.

Under these circumstances, the nursing home that retains its help for long periods of time is obviously paying a competitive wage, has good working conditions and is delivering decent care to its residents. It is one sign of a quality nursing home if the staff members you speak with have been there for several years.

TALK TO SOME OF THE STAFF

If at all possible, attempt to talk to nursing staff members on the individual units. The answers to some of these questions might be very revealing:

1. How much overtime do you work? Is it mandatory? How do you feel when you have to work overtime?
2. Do you like working here? Why?
3. Why did you choose geriatric nursing?
4. When do you restrain patients?
5. How would you characterize the nurse–doctor relationship?

CHAPTER 5

EVALUATING A NURSING HOME

OBTAINING A LIST

Since the telephone directory is ambiguous, and county medical societies or departments of aging will only provide lists of all homes in a given geographical area, it is suggested that initial inquiries begin with your medical contacts. Doctors in family practice, orthopedic physicians or gerontologists will have some familiarity with nursing homes in your area. Hospital discharge planners, medical social workers or visiting nurses also deal with nursing homes on a continuing basis and are an excellent source for compiling your initial list.

Because so many nursing home patients suffer from Alzheimer's disease, it is recommended that contact be made with the local chapter of the Alzheimer's Association. This organization, with a national headquarters at 70 East Lake Street, Chicago, IL, 60601, has very active local and state chapters which can provide a great deal of useful information to families of patients with that affliction.

Family friends and acquaintances who have already chosen a home are an obvious source of candid information. It may sound macabre, but checking the obituaries in local newspapers can be a useful tool. The survivors of the elderly who have recently died in a nursing home will often have strong feelings about the facility of their choice, and are usually willing to share this information after an appropriate time has elapsed.

After a list of facilities has been collected from several sources, the names should be compared and a final list made from those duplications that appear. It is suggested that initial investigation begin with names listed by two or more sources.

EVALUATING A NURSING HOME*

The following lists of questions form a detailed evaluation constructed in an attempt to alert the investigator to many areas of potential problems. It is designed with the assumption that the potential resident will have a stay of not less than 30 days and possibly several years. It considers the patient's movement as at least partially restricted, and that therefore small details of physical environment can make a large difference in the resident's quality of life. The evaluation is a guide of what to look for and what questions to ask.

It has already been suggested that an investigation begin with medicare/medicaid licensed homes. With this prerequisite, it is not necessary to check many details, such as the number of fire doors** or proper licensing of personnel.

A careful review of the items listed is recommended. It is not necessary to answer each and every question.

EXTERIOR

Are there wheelchair access ramps and handrails?
Are the grounds and walks well maintained without clutter?
Is there a protected outside area with lawn furniture?
If the weather and time are appropriate are residents outside?
Bird feeders and seasonal plantings would be thoughtful. Do any appear?

HALLS AND LOBBY

Are the halls well lit?
Are there handrails in the corridors?
Are the halls wide enough for two wheelchairs to pass?
Is the housekeeping adequate?
Are the furnishings well maintained and adequate?
Are the exits well marked and not locked?

---

* Note: The list of questions in this section is designed primarily for skilled nursing home facilities for the aged. The questions are valid for custodial facilities although they have less licensed personnel and rehabilitation functions.

** A careful review of news clippings concerning nursing home fires reveals that although headlined in the newspaper as such, they are usually fires in custodial or board and care facilities. These institutions usually had smoke detectors, but through loopholes in state regulations did not have sprinkler systems. No recent fatalities have been reported in nursing homes that had sprinkler systems.

Are safety devices such as fire extinguishers visible?
Are there sufficient elevators for the number of patients?
Are the elevators large enough for wheelchairs?
Are the laundry and food carts in the halls covered?
Are residents allowed free access throughout the facility?
Are state licenses on display?
Is there a bulletin board indicating recent and future events?
Are safety precautions taken during mopping and waxing?
Are the halls cluttered?
Are old cooking smells evident?
Are there other stale odors?
Is there a cover–up smell of disinfectant?
Are residents ambulating in the halls and common areas?
Is any carpeting too thick for walkers or wheelchairs?

RESIDENT ROOMS

Look at more than one room and more than one unit.
Do semi–private accommodations have more than the two recommended
   beds?
Other than the hospital bed, can residents provide their own furniture?
Is there a privacy curtain for each bed?
Is each resident area at least 80 square feet?
Is each bed at least four feet from another bed?
Does the room have a dresser, mirror and closet space?
Are a bedside table and overhead light provided?
Is there a moisture–proof mattress?
Are mattresses covered with protective devices?
If the call bell becomes disconnected does it ring the nurse?
Can a private phone be installed?
Can pictures be hung on the walls?
Is there one comfortable chair for each resident?
Is there fresh drinking water with a glass by each bed?
What is the policy on room transfers?
Does each patient involved have to agree on a transfer?
Do the television sets have earphones?
Is there room for easy wheelchair access?
Does each room have a thermostat set on 72°?
If the room does not have an air–conditioner, can you install your own?
May residents smoke in their rooms? If not, are there designated smoking
   areas?
Are smoking areas well maintained and supervised?
Are ashtrays plentiful, clean and well placed?

RESIDENT'S BATH

The bath should not be shared by more than four persons.
Are there call bells near the toilet, sink and tub?
Are there grab bars at the toilet and tub/shower?
Does the tub/shower have a non–skid bottom?
Is the bath large enough for easy wheelchair access?
Are raised toilet seats available?
Is the bathroom clean and odor free?
Are there filled soap and paper towel dispensers?

DINING FACILITIES

Is the menu rotated on at least a three week cycle?
Does the posted menu agree with what is actually served?
Are the dishes and utensils appropriate for the patient's ability?
(Dishes and utensils should not be paper or plastic unless the patient is
    on precautions because of contagion.)
Is the dining room easily accessible by wheelchair?
Are aides readily available to help those who have difficulty?
Are dining room personnel trained in the Heimlich maneuver?
Is adequate time given to those who need time with their meal?
Are meals served at rational times or for staff's convenience?
There should not be more than 14 hours between meals.
Is care taken with seatmate assignments?

FOOD

Is the food tasty, warm and attractively presented?
Is the food warm and covered when served in the patient's room?
Is there an alternate entree for the main meal?
Are snacks and beverages served between meals?
Is care taken in the preparation of special diets?
Are fresh fruits and vegetables served in season?
Are the servings prepackaged or cooked from scratch?

RESIDENT ACTIVITIES

Does the facility have a trained recreation director?
Are the recreational areas of sufficient size?
Is there a recreational calendar posted that seems adequate?
Do these events really occur?
Are there activities for residents of different abilities?
Are there activities for residents of divergent interests?

Are special events planned for holidays?
Are wheelchair patients transported to outside activities?
Are religious services available?
Are hobby and game equipment available (kilns, board games, etc.)?
Is there a library with current books and periodicals?
Are large print materials available?
Is newspaper delivery available?
Does the local library have bookmobile service?
Will volunteers obtain books for patients?
Is there transportation to events outside the facility?

Nursing Care

Are the aides certified by the state?
If they are not, is there an in–house training program?
Is there in–service training for the nursing staff?
Is a nursing care plan prepared for each patient on admission?
Do the staff emphasize activities for daily living (ADLs)?
Is a licensed nurse on duty for each unit 24 hours a day?
Is the facility fully staffed or does the facility use pool (outside temporary
   help) nurses and aides?
What's the average job tenure for nurses and aides?
Are nurses or aides allowed to turn off call bells at the nursing station?
   A definite no–no.
What is each unit's staffing for each shift?
Are bedridden patients turned and repositioned every two hours?
Are physical restraints checked every two hours and the patient checked
   for friction marks and toileted or changed?
Is the staff attitude toward patients condescending or impatient?
Does the staff seem to congregate constantly at the nurses' station or in
   the employees' lounge?
Does the staff interact pleasantly with the patients?
Does the staff do a complete change for an incontinent patient?
Does the administration allow you to speak freely with the staff?
Does the staff attempt bladder retraining?
Is the staff truly interested in rehabilitation or does their attitude seem
   more custodial?

Medical Services

Does the patient's present doctor have privileges?
If not, who will be the patient's doctor?
What hospital does the home use in an emergency?
Does the patient's doctor have privileges there?

What ambulance service does the home use and what is its response time?
Does the ambulance service have trained Emergency Medical Technicians (EMTs)?
Is a doctor on call 24 hours a day?
Are specialists available (e.g., orthopedic doctors, etc.)?
Will the patient have a physical at the time of admission?
Can you use your own pharmacy?
If not, will the pharmacy the facility uses fill prescriptions generically?
Will the doctor see the patient *at least once every 30 days* for the first 90 days?
Is a separate examination room available?
Are suction machines, oxygen and other equipment available?
What are the qualifications of the medical director?
How many other facilities does he serve?
Does the medical director have a financial interest in the facility?

THE RESIDENTS

Are the residents neat and are their nails trimmed?
Are the men shaven?
Are the women neat and their hair well kept?
Are confused patients up and dressed?
Do an excessive number of patients seem physically restrained?
Are many patients lethargic (a sign of chemical restraint)?
Are most patients dressed in clothes rather than gowns?
Are the patients hesitant to speak with you?
Are the patients interacting with each other?
Do they seem to like the nursing home?

GENERAL

Is there a patient's resident council?
Is there a patient's family council?
Were you given a copy of the Patient's Bill of Rights?
Can a spouse of a patient or lovers have privacy if they wish?
Are social workers available?
Are visiting hours extensive?
Are children allowed to visit?
Are pets allowed to be brought in?
Is alcohol permitted with a doctor's order?
Is the ''no tipping'' rule enforced?
Does the facility have a problem with theft?

OTHER SERVICES

Are hairdressing and haircuts available on a regular basis?
How often is personal laundry picked up and delivered?
Are the appropriate therapists available?
Are the therapy rooms fully equipped and utilized?
Are there regular visits by an optometrist?
Are there regular visits by a podiatrist?
Is a dentist available?
Can X-rays be taken at the facility?

FINANCIAL QUESTIONS

Is a contract required and can you have a copy to study?
How much deposit is required?
When is the balance of the deposit returned on the patient's discharge?
What is the basic daily rate and exactly what does it include?
How much are other services such as:

> Laundry
> Beautician or barber
> Podiatrist
> Therapists
> Pharmacy (based on drugs presently prescribed)
> Minor medical items such as laxatives, tissues, etc.
> Major medical items such as walkers, wheelchairs, etc.

Does the facility charge extra for special nursing such as incontinence care, feeding or other services?
How are the residents' valuables such as jewelry handled?
What happens if the patient's funds should be depleted and it is necessary to apply for Title XIX (Medicaid)?

THE WAITING LIST
(WHERE APPLICABLE)

How long is the waiting list?
What is the approximate wait?
What is the *exact* procedure to get placed on the list?
Does the facility give preference to hospital transfers or other medical conditions?
Does the facility have any special units the potential patient might qualify for?
If a bed is turned down, can the patient's name be retained high on the list and for what length of time?

It is a long list of questions for a difficult job, but there is something cathartic about a thorough and diligent nursing home search. Following this list you will know you have done the best to assure the patient's well–being.

You Have Found the Right Nursing Home but There Are No Vacancies

In some areas of the country, such as in the Northeast, there is an acute shortage of nursing home beds. The states in which this situation exists have attacked the problem in several ways. Some states require that medical profiles of potential residents be prepared, and have devised rating systems for the amount of nursing care individuals require according to these profiles. Waiting lists are then prepared based on the rated need for skilled care. Some of the other states have mandated the sanctity of the waiting list. In these instances, the nursing homes must accept patients strictly according to their placement on the list.

The procedure in any given state can be determined by speaking with the State Department of Health, hospital discharge planners, medical social workers, county medical societies or physicians whose practice includes the elderly.

Certain financial abuses have occurred in those areas with nursing home bed shortages. Either through dishonest staff members or rapacious owners, some nursing homes have requested special gratuities, endowments or gifts to facilitate admission. In most jurisdictions this practice is considered to be exactly what it is: a payoff. It can result in heavy fines, criminal prosecution or loss of licensure.

Medicaid reimbursement rates are far less than what a nursing home can charge a self–pay patient, and often these rates are below the institution's cost. As a general rule nursing homes will do all they can to give preference to the self–pay resident admission. Toward this end, homes will often require extensive financial information on the application form, large deposits or illegally attempt to get guarantees of payment by family members. In those states with mandated waiting lists nursing homes will refuse to take potential Medicaid patients or enter them onto the waiting list until the individual has been formally accepted into the Medicaid program, a bureaucratic process that can take weeks, if not months.

Anticipation

Logically anticipating the future and making a potential nursing home placement decision in advance is the surest method to overcome the waiting list problem. Several chronic diseases in the elderly have predictable lag time before skilled nursing care is required. The natural course of a disease of this sort progressively renders a patient with worsening disability. Patients with Alzheimer's disease, even though their home care is presently adequate, should be placed on the waiting list of the appropriate nursing home. Unfortunately, almost every Alzheimer's patient will eventually require skilled nursing care. Therefore it is suggested that the name of the patient be placed on the waiting list once this dementia has been diagnosed.

In most instances, if a patient's name rotates to the top of a list and a bed is offered and declined, the name can still remain high on the list for future consideration. In cases where available funds are not adequate to cover potential nursing home costs, a Medicaid application can be instituted and finalized in advance, if the decision is properly anticipated.

CHECK ON SPECIAL UNITS

A particular nursing home might have a long waiting list, but it also may have a specialized unit, such as an Alzheimer's or orthopedic unit. These nursing homes are permitted to jump names on their waiting lists in order to select patients for their empty beds in these specialized units.

FILE THE APPLICATION

A telephone call to a nursing home to place a name on their waiting list is not adequate. Although a listing of these telephone inquiries may be kept, selections will be made using the waiting list developed by applications on file. Nursing home applications are often long and personal, and contain intimate financial and medical data. They are onerous to fill out, but are a necessity if you wish to be seriously considered.

CHAPTER 6

ADMISSION

HOW TO PREPARE THE
NEW RESIDENT

BEFORE THE ADMISSION

A diligent search has been made, several nursing homes have been investigated and a final choice has been made. Admission procedures and arrangements have been completed. The day of transfer approaches. The soon-to-be patient, perhaps a surviving parent, becomes increasingly agitated as the day of admission nears. Perhaps her attitude corresponds to this case:

Mary H., 85

Mary H. lived independently for 20 years after her husband's death. Her major medical problem was Parkinson's disease, a progressive disorder of the brain leading to a resting tremor of the hand, dysfunctional gait and occasionally cognitive deterioration. In Mary's case, she lost the ability to wash dishes, to prepare food, to clean her apartment, to groom herself and ultimately to walk. As her ability to cope with simple daily activities and chores worsened, she and her son discussed her moving into his condominium. Her son hired a homemaker to assist his mother during the day. He found that providing her care in the evening and night consumed all of his free time. They reached a mutual agreement to investigate nursing homes. Three local nursing homes were thoroughly investigated. Mary was taken to the one her son considered best in order to obtain her final approval. She enjoyed the staff and felt comfortable at the nursing home. They mutually agreed to file an application.

Mary's transfer from her own apartment to her son's condominium had been traumatic enough, and the possibility of another radical change truly frightened her. She became increasingly depressed as her admission day approached. Her usually placid personality abruptly changed as she verbally lashed out at her family.

"You want to get rid of me!" she announced out of context at dinner one night.

"No, I don't, Mother," her son answered her quietly.

"That home will take what little money I have left, but you don't care. You want me dead!"

Her son was alarmed and confused at this outburst. He began to propitiate Mary, and canceled the admission to everyone's later regret.

Mary's case is a typical example of last minute resistance to the nursing home admission. She had lost the resiliency of youth which permits facile adaptation to abrupt changes in life. Her recent move from her own home to her son's was emotionally catastrophic, and she found it difficult to contemplate another change. Although she participated in the nursing home decision, she had strong second thoughts. She felt rejected, and perceived that her final place in society had been wrenched away, taking with it her last vestige of independence. She was also worried about finances, which is almost a universal fear among the elderly, regardless of the extent of their assets.

One usual pre–admission dilemma was not present in Mary's case. Residents who go directly from their own home to a nursing home face the prospect of leaving behind most of their cherished belongings, pets and friends. This anticipated loss often impedes the nursing home transfer and admission.

As the admission day approaches, the patient's family may find themselves experiencing profound relief. This is a common reaction, for there is a great deal of concern over the patient's care and well–being. This feeling of relief can be internally misunderstood and cause family members to doubt their motives. They begin to wonder why they look toward the admission date with a sense of impending freedom, and view it as a welcome event. Second thoughts arise with these questions: Have we done the right thing? Has our decision been made with love? Are we negating our responsiblity? Are we dumping a member of our own family? It is from within these concerns that the seeds of guilt flourish.

The family must understand that their *relief should not cause guilt*. The family, as the solider in combat, has been going through an emotionally trying time, and has had to deal with difficult inner feelings. It would be unnatural not to feel relief as the emotional conflict draws to a close.

Human decisions are often reached in a passive manner. A choice to change life's direction may not be reached by a careful weighing of alternatives, but by the thrust of events which force us into a certain course of action. If mutual family decisions are usually reached in this manner, and the nursing home decision has been arrived at by circumstances rather than choice, the family must be careful not to resort to the "social lie." The family that operates in this manner may often lie to the prospective patient when they protest.

"Don't worry, Mom, you'll only be in that place for a week . . . you'll only be in that place until we get back from Florida . . . you'll only be in that place until we get your room redone . . . until your hip recovers . . . until you get your strength back . . ." How many are the countless variations?

Such avoidance, such postponement of unpleasantries, will only complicate the patient's admission and may very well make the final accommodation to the nursing home impossible. It is guaranteed that the social lie told today to avoid a small amount of pain will cause untold grief when the situation must be refaced.

PROPERTY PREPARATION

Most nursing homes will allow their patients to bring a certain amount of personal belongings in addition to clothing and toiletries. The hospital bed cannot be replaced as it has side rails that may be needed, is of a height that is convenient for transfers and can be raised or lowered sectionally into a variety of useful positions. Most facilities will also require that the side table remain, as it is needed to hold medications. The over–the–bed–table is another standard piece of furniture that should not be removed. Bureaus, bookcases, a personal easy chair and wall hangings are usually allowed. We encourage residents to decorate their rooms with as many personal items as possible.

Framed photographs are important, as is the photo album which can revive past memories. A few personal items can transform an otherwise sterile hospital–like room into a place of familiarity.

The following items are recommended:

A *recliner* to replace the room's side chair. If cost is no object, a recliner that aids in standing is useful for many patients.

A *VCR* can act as a surrogate visitor, in addition to its ordinary entertainment features, if faraway relatives prepare tapes of significant family events.

An *AM-FM radio with earplugs* can be protection for the resident whose rommate watches annoying television programs. This radio can also be played at anytime day or night without disturbing other patients.

All possessions taken to the nursing home should be inventoried and marked with the patient's name.

For patients who are legally blind or who have other types of handicaps that make it impossible for them to hold or to turn book pages, the talking book program is a godsend. This free program provides a cassette player or phonograph and tapes that can be chosen trom hundreds of selections. The tapes are returned to a regional center in the mailers provided and new tapes are mailed out the day their request is received. To obtain these services contact your state library or The Library for the Blind and Handicapped, a division of the Library of Congress, Washington, D.C.

CLOTHING

The importance of proper clothing and footwear for the nursing home resident is crucial. These people are not at a resort hotel or on a cruise ship. They are the elderly who for one or more reasons cannot live independently or with home care aid. They may have chronic disorders, a poor sense of balance or any other number of major or minor medical disorders. Nearly 72% of nursing home residents need some help in dressing. Those with poor balance should be able to dress themselves while sitting. A large percentage of nursing home patients are incontinent, and the selection of proper clothing for those individuals is extremely important.

Clothing should be of materials that are easily laundered, and made of fabrics that are not irritating to the delicate skin of the elderly. The items taken should be selected with safety in mind, which discourages long robes which might cause people to trip, or footwear with heels of any height. The clothing should be easy to put on. Big buttons are more easily managed than small, front buttons more accessible than rear and simple buckles or Velcro fasteners are the easiest of all. Fasteners on the front side of a garment are convenient. Underwear should be of soft and absorbent material.

The safest shoes with the most support have tie laces and broad heels. Floppy slippers without support should not be taken. Cotton socks that can be frequently changed and can absorb perspiration should be included. Socks should fit loosely. The use of garters or rolling and twisting stockings to keep them up will hinder circulation.

Physiological changes in the elderly affect how comfortable they are in various types of clothing material. Wool, for example, irritates the thinner and dryer skin of the aging. Cotton brushed nylon and acrylic velour are comfortable fabrics, while stiff cloth such as denim and heavy linen will be uncomfortable for the elderly. Fabrics such as mohair can irritate if there is inhalation of the filaments. Nylon pajamas or nightdress will make turning over in bed easier.

It will help patients with restricted joint motion to have light garments with large front openings and easy to use fasteners. Trousers with a stretch waist and full hips are more easily donned by the restricted male.

As we know, the elderly often feel chilly. However, heavy clothing will restrict movement and be difficult to put on and take off. Several layers of light clothing are recommended. A lightweight cardigan sweater will be more comfortable than a heavy jacket.

It is often possible to modify the patient's present clothing by the use of Velcro tape or replacing small buttons with large ones. Clothing adaptation or special clothing can be of considerable importance to the patient's sense of well–being and pride. The incontinent resident, with clothing cut up the back or held with a Velcro fastener, will have a greater sense of self worth if he is dressed rather than perpetually confined to wearing a johnny gown. Unless directly asked, the staff may not raise this subject in advance, and therefore these clothing needs should be anticipated by the patient's family.

Many of the larger nursing homes in metropolitan areas actually have fashion shows where mature models present special need clothing and sales representatives are present to take orders. A medical supply house can be contacted to see if they provide this type of clothing, or if they do not, to recommend a source. Sears publishes the *Sears Home Health Care Catalog*, and this can be obtained by writing to the Sears Tower, Chicago, IL, 60684. The nursing home social worker or occupational therapist may also be able to provide catalogs or suggestions.

All clothing should be marked and inventoried before the patient is admitted.

THE DAY OF ADMISSION

The first day of a nursing home admission is not the last time the family will see the patient. It is not necessary to make a grand outing of the occasion, or to have a large group accompany the patient. A mid–morning arrival is suggested, with not more than two people accompanying the patient.

A nursing home adjustment is difficult enough at best and a tearful scene at the time of admission is hardly conducive to an orderly and placid transition.

Plan to spend several hours on that first day. There will be more paperwork to be done, no matter how thorough the prior preparation. It is also important to help the new resident arrange his personal belongings and meet the roommate, and you should introduce yourself to the unit nursing staff.

Some nursing homes will take great care in attempting to assign roommates of mutual age and interests. Other facilities, perhaps because of a shortage of available beds, will have little opportunity to arrange a thoughtful pairing. The roommate relationship can be one of the most important factors in the early transition to the nursing home milieu. This adjustment can be difficult, but sharing a room with a confused resident who talks loudly and constantly in strange non sequiturs will only complicate the situation. Bizarre as it may sound, sharing a room with a comatose patient or an advanced stage Alzheimer's patient will provide an element of quiet for the patient who desires privacy but who does not have a private room.

Unhappy roommates are a constant cause of friction in nursing homes. Most facilities will arrange room transfers providing all the residents involved are in agreement.

HUMANIZE THE NEW PATIENT TO THE STAFF

If you are able to personalize the new patient to the staff as an individual rather than just another new admission, the first important step in assuring good care has been taken. The staff, in this instance, consists of those on the unit such as the charge nurse, the floor nurses and the nursing assistants (aides). A few appropriate remarks such as, "She is the mother of six . . . she taught English for 30 years . . . a person who truly loves music . . . mother was born in the old country . . ." or any other item of interest or importance to the patient's personality will help invoke feeling in the staff. They will begin to think of the patient as a person rather than as the second bed in room 202.

The staff also needs to know the patient's large and small personal idiosyncrasies. Even minor items of preference such as the desire for a night light, or the dislike of a particular newspaper, can make a difference in adjustment. The staff should also be made aware of the new resident's:

Degree of mobility: walks with canes, needs wheelchair, etc.
Ability with activities for daily living (more of these later)
Special hobbies or interests
Dietary preferences

Remember, these are the people who will spend 24 hours a day with the patient. The more they can consider the patient as a full person, the better their interaction.

Violet R., 76

Violet was admitted to a skilled nursing home directly from a custodial facility. She suffered from Alzheimer's disease and was uncommunicative, spoke in word salad and had a flat affect, which meant that she showed no emotion. There was no family member present at the time of admission. Violet rapidly began to deteriorate physically. After several weeks a cousin arrived at the nursing home for a visit and casually mentioned to a member of the staff that in her younger years Violet had been a concert cellist.

Social Services immediately obtained a tape player and tapes of classical chamber music which they placed by Violet's bed. Violet registered her first emotion when she heard the opening bars of a Mozart cello concerto. Complete rehabilitation was not possible with this irreversible disease, but rudimentary communication was established, and Violet's quality of life certainly improved.

GIVE A TRUE ASSESSMENT

Any attempt to hide the new resident's cognitive and physical shortcomings will mislead the staff and be a disservice to the patient. It is preferable that the nursing personnel know the complete limitations of the new resident so they can plan and treat accordingly, rather than hear a sanitized version based on family hope more than reality.

TALK WITH THE CHARGE NURSE

If the facility has 60 beds or less, arrange a meeting with the director of nursing. We tend to feel that nursing homes larger than this preclude the DN from having direct patient contact, and in that instance it is recommended that a conversation be held with the unit's *day charge nurse.*

It is during this conversation that you should inquire as to what special equipment might be either useful or necessary for the patient. For example, a reclining cardiac chair is useful for some patients, and this item is usually not standard equipment in the average nursing home. The nurse can give you advice on these matters and suggest either where to buy or rent this type of equipment.

ACTIVITIES OF DAILY LIVING

It is also during this conversation that the subject of activities of daily living (ADLs) should be discussed in depth. You should be prepared to inform the nurse to what extent the patient can perform the following personal care tasks:

Bathing	Transfer/bed/chair	Walk/need help
Toileting	Teeth and mouth care	Shaving
Comb hair	Wash hair	Nail care
Feet care	Dressing	Eating

After considering your comments, the nurse may decide to have an assessment by the occupational and physical therapists to determine if rehabilitative training is indicated.

If you have selected your nursing home correctly, the staff should be interested in increasing or at least maintaining the level of functioning ADLs within the limits of the patient's ability.

The poor facility, or the one with an acute staff shortage, will skimp on the time necessary to maintain or increase ADLs. As has been stated earlier, it is far easier for the harried aide to dress a patient than it is to stand by while a resident with restricted mobility fumbles with clothing. The patient should not only be allowed, but actively encouraged to perform as many self–care tasks as possible. Failure to adhere to this precept can only result in the loss of function. If the recent transfer was due to a new disability, retraining might be necessary.

In the case of an incontinent patient, bladder retraining might be considered, or if this is not practical, the use of special clothing and absorbent pads should be discussed at this meeting.

It is important that the degree of impairment be outlined for the patient who has elements of confusion or short term memory loss. The nurse needs to know if this confusion had an acute onset, which might be due to a recent medical condition or drug reaction. The staff also needs to know if the confusion has been progressive. Some patients will exhibit mild confusion, but only at certain times such as awakening in the middle of the night. This would be an important factor for nurses to consider when tending to that resident's nightly needs.

PATIENT CARE PLAN

The importance of this initial discussion with the charge nurse is fundamental because shortly after admission the **Patient Care Plan** will be prepared. This nursing plan is usually an interdisciplinary function, with input by the nursing department, the appropriate therapists and the dietitian. This plan, in conjunction with the physician's **Plan of Medical Care,** indicates the care to be given and the goals to be accomplished, as well as which professional service is responsible for the delivery of each element.

TALK WITH THE DOCTOR

If a full physical examination has not been given to the patient in the very recent past, one will be performed shortly after admission by her doctor or the medical director. It is important for you to know the results of this physical, and to understand fully the patient's present physical and mental condition along with overall prognosis.

Understand exactly what drugs have been ordered, what they are for and any probable side effects they may have. This is the time to find out what treatments and therapies have been ordered by the **Plan of Medical Care.** If the patient is confused, ask about your physician's position on physical and chemical restraints as they pertain to this care.

Physicians develop a problem list, the foundation of the Plan of Medical Care, for each patient and record it in the record. Each problem is listed in rank order; thus, problem one is the most active or serious. A medical plan is constructed for each problem. We recommend that you ask the physician to discuss the patient's problem list with you. During this conversation, you should learn what the medical conditions are and their respective treatments and prognosis.

If the prognosis is poor, it is best to understand the full ramifications of the patient's condition. It is not unusual to see the families of a deteriorating patient insist on therapies that are not only useless for rehabilitation, but uncomfortable and painful for the patient. It is best to deal with these questions honestly, and consider the patient's comfort if rehabilitation is not possible.

Sometimes the patient's physical condition is stable and treatments are designed to maintain functional equilibrium for as long as possible. In this instance, improvement is unlikely, and this must be understood. We are often inured by the media to expect miracles. Although the young may often bounce back from devastating disabilities, the elderly rarely make such rapid and dynamic improvements.

A positive attitude and will to overcome are powerful healing tools for the elderly. It is not uncommon to see two patients suffering from a similar type of stroke enter a nursing home at the same time. One patient, with a positive mental approach, is retrained, makes physical adjustments and returns home as a functioning individual. The second, with a negative and defeatist attitude, shows little interest in rehabilitation, undergoes little physical improvement and eventually begins to withdraw. Medically each person was treated similarly, yet desire and motivation made the difference for recovery.

The nursing home elderly have not only suffered the losses inherent in life's last cycle, but they have been removed from normal society and placed in a custodial setting. It is often simple for many of them to slide into "institutionalization" with all the negative aspects of that type of mental attitude. It is incumbent on the residents' advocates, family and friends, to extend a support network as far as possible in order to retain the necessary contact with outside life.

SELECT A PATIENT'S ADVOCATE

Before proceeding to the next steps concerning the new nursing home resident, if the family and friends have not already done so, they must select one person to be the **patient's advocate.** This is the single individual who should be responsible for monitoring care, both with doctors and nurses, and the liaison with the nursing home administration. The advocate should undertake any other functions necessary for the well–being of the resident.

Physicians do not have the time nor inclination to answer identical questions from a host of well meaning family, nor will the nursing staff be responsive to a group of complainers on the patient's behalf. One person should be responsible for all official contact with medical, accounting or other personnel.

It should be the responsibility of this individual to understand the patient's medical condition completely, as well as the therapies and medications involved and the prognosis. It is this person who will closely monitor the patient's care and take necessary steps if it proves inadequate.

CHAPTER 7

THE FOLLOW-UP

MONITORING THE NURSING HOME PATIENT

THE PERIOD OF ADJUSTMENT

The first 90 days are critical!

These first weeks in a nursing home are not only a difficult emotional adjustment, but can be so traumatic for the elderly as to increase their death rate. Studies have shown that those at greatest risk are the severely depressed, the highly anxious, the intermittently confused and those over 85. Reducing relocation impact begins with the patient's participation in the nursing home decision, and continues with the mutual support of family and staff after admission.

Because of the emotional and physical danger to the elderly during periods of transition, change should be kept to a minimum when possible. Future anticipation is once again important. If a patient is admitted to a custodial type facility with a deteriorating medical condition, it may be possible to predict that at some future point that individual will require skilled nursing care. In cases of this nature, it is recommended that initial placement be in a facility that has both levels of care. When the day arrives when skilled care is needed, the resident may need to only change floors and rooms rather than transfer to a new nursing home. The surroundings would still be familiar, the transition softened and the trauma involved reduced to a minimum.

Experienced geriatric personnel have a saying: "She turned to the wall." They have seen this displayed countless times as highly depressed patients simply withdraw from all social contact into an inner cocoon. Unless there is drug and psychotherapeutic intervention, and this is not always successful, death usually follows shortly.

There is no way to emphasize more strongly the importance of the transition period than to state that the patient's life may depend on it going as smoothly as possible.

HONESTY

This is the time for more honesty with the new resident. The patient may be visibly upset and beg family and friends to take her home. **Do not lie!** Do not tell her that you will bring her home next Tuesday in order to calm her temporarily and allow the visit to proceed. Social lies of this nature may get family members through an emotional visit, but it only prolongs the transition period and inhibits adjustment.

Do not be surprised if a difficult and unhappy new resident has a host of complaints that may not be true. The depressed new resident will often describe the nursing home and its staff in a manner which compares it unfavorably with a medieval dungeon. She may say that the food is moldy, the help sadistic and the roommate has all the attributes of Rasputin. Take note of such complaints, but in the beginning it is suggested that you discuss them at length with the staff in order to make a personal determination as to their validity.

The transition period is characterized by intense feelings of isolation and abandonment. Patients fear that no one will listen to them. They worry that their concerns will not be seriously heeded. Listen to them and keep track of their feelings. This is the time to work through negative perceptions engendered by entrance into an institution. Through availability and listening, you can provide more therapy than any medicine their physicians can prescribe.

Excessive demands placed on nursing home staff are telltale signs of guilt–related feelings. A good staff will recognize the true messages underpinning a demanding patient or family's motives and will offer assistance in working through these feelings. However, most nurses and aides feel antagonized by the difficult and demanding patient and family and react by delaying response time, delivering incomplete care or returning antagonism.

NURSES AND AIDES ARE NOT MAIDS

Some patients and families, all too aware of the high cost of nursing home care, expect nursing home personnel to provide personalized services: to wait on them. This is not the function of professional people except as medically indicated. It is also contrary to good nursing practice. Patients should be expected to do all they can for themselves. They should be highly encouraged to perform activities of daily living. Residents and families who are insistent on the performance of small services will not only disrupt the unit, but will create a negative attitude toward the patient.

These excessive demands in the case of patients are an expression of their fear of abandonment and need for attention of any sort.

TIME

WHAT'S IMPORTANT TO THE PATIENTS

In 1989 Rosalie A. Kane, a Social Worker at the University of Minnesota, conducted a study in 45 nursing homes concerning the everyday choices that patients were most concerned about. To everyone's surprise, except the patients, those concerns were ranked as follows:

1. Going out—leave the home to walk, shop, etc.
2. Phones and mail—contacts with families and friends.
3. Roommates—having a choice of roommates.
4. Care—routines requiring aid, such as bathing.
5. Activities—recreation, entertainment and crafts.
6. Food—type of food, mealtimes and being fed.
7. Money—access to and control of funds.
8. Getting up—when and if to get up in the morning.
9. Going to bed—when to go to bed at night.
10. Visitors—which guests come and when they come.

A TYPICAL NURSING HOME SCHEDULE

The Kane study indicates that control of time and such basic decisions as when to get up and when to go to bed are among the primary concerns of nursing home residents. This desire for independence is often in conflict with the day-to-day functioning of the nursing home, which is an institution designed to dispense food, housekeeping and health care. By its very nature, the facility must operate on a rather strict schedule, which intrudes upon its residents' independence. In order to place this in perspective, following is reproduced a typical nursing home day:

DAY SHIFT (7:00 A.M. to 3:00 P.M.)

7:30 — Breakfast (often served in room)
8:00 — Dress, patient care or self-care   Medications
10:00 — Snacks and nourishment
           1st recreation period
           Church services on Thursday (rotating denominations)
12:00 — Dinner (Main meal of the day)   Medications

1:30 — 2nd recreation period
3:00 — Snacks and nourishment

EVENING SHIFT (3:00 P.M. to 11:00 P.M.)

4:00 — Medications
5:00 — Supper
8:00 — Snacks and nourishment   Medications
9:00 — Preparation for bed

Visiting hours are usually from 10:00 A.M. to 8:00 P.M. each day. Individual therapies are scheduled throughout the day. Hairdressers, barbers, dentists and podiatrists are seen by appointment. Each resident is scheduled for one bath a week except for self–care patients. As will be mentioned later, more frequent complete bathing of the elderly is not recommended.

Shift times may vary slightly among facilities, but the schedule listed is typical.

NURSES REPORT

This occurs at shift change and is when the charge nurse informs the incoming shift of any significant information concerning the patients' conditions. This interchange usually takes from 10 to 15 minutes, and it is a poor time to attempt to speak with the charge nurse.

STRUCTURED TIME

At a cursory glance, the schedule might appear rather stark. The schedule is an attempt to balance three conflicting needs: the necessity to provide maximum utilization of staff, the need for a loose but definite structure to the day, and a desire to allow freedom of choice for the resident as much as possible. While the elderly rightfully resent being told when to arise and when to prepare for bed, they also have a definite need for routine and a structured day. They wish to have recreational activities available, but do not want bubbly social directors pulling them from their room to participate. Residents like to have hairdressing appointments on a given day at a given time, while also having the opportunity to watch a favorite soap opera at another hour.

RECREATIONAL PROGRAMS

Popular recreational programs are bingo, word games and card games. Television watching is popular, and most nursing homes schedule VCR movies in the lounge several times a week. Some patients form their own card partnerships for regular games of set back, canasta and bridge. Most institutions also schedule special events for holidays, birthdays and other special occasions.

RESIDENT COUNCILS

Most nursing homes have an elected Resident Council which meets to discuss matters of policy and acts as a forum for complaints between patients and the administration. They usually spend most of their time talking about food.

Many nursing homes also have Resident Family Councils which function in the same manner as the Resident Councils. The accomplishments of both groups are completely dependent on the strength and will of their leading members. Generally speaking, the Family Council can swing more weight with the administration.

LIQUOR AND SEX

Moderate amounts of liquor can be dispensed to a resident upon a doctor's order. A certain number of nonprofit homes with fundamentalist religious orientations may not allow this, while other facilities will hold weekly "socials" where mild alcoholic beverages are served. Smoking may not be allowed in a resident's room, and this is dependent on local fire laws and the occupant's mental clarity. Designated smoking areas are usually provided. However, many states are legislating laws which make all health institutions "smoke free."

The Patient's Bill of Rights guarantees privacy to each individual, and this includes the privacy of spouses and lovers. There does seem to be prejudice by staff members toward the elderly indulging in sexual intercourse, but the facility has an obligation to permit such consensual activity.

PRIVATE DUTY HELP

The staff of most nursing homes is usually pleased to see private duty help hired by the patient or family. This not only relieves personnel from providing care for the patient, but it also means that nurses and aides do not have to make periodic checks on that patient while the private duty help is there. Private duty offers one-on-one attention, and can be of immense help if care such as ambulation is necessary. The hiring of aides is adequate for most functions requiring personal care and attention, while, obviously, licensed personnel must be obtained if nursing treatments are to be performed.

Private duty care will cost between 10 and 25 dollars an hour, depending on license and geographic area. Often a split-shift person is available, and even three or four hours of one–on–one care can be beneficial. In terminal cases, changes of position, sponge baths, rub downs, sips of water and conversation can go far to make the patient more comfortable.

Family members or a hired "sitter" who need not be trained can help the patient in certain instances within limitations. In the case of a confused patient who may be a wanderer, a sitter can keep watch. Her presence might be enough to stop the wandering and so keep the patient from being subject to unwanted chemical or physical restraints. Although the sitter's authority to intervene would be limited she could alert the staff if necessary. People hired for this function can be obtained for less money than trained or licensed personnel.

THE MONITORING VISIT

Shortly after the patient's admission it is time to begin a follow–up on the care and the facility. This cannot all be accomplished in a single visit, as careful observation must be made over a period of time.

THE MONITORING VISIT RULES

If you consistently visit every Sunday at 2:00, you may rest assured that the patient will always be up, dressed and well taken care of every Sunday at 1:45. Occasionally *vary your visiting hours.*

The day shift may be great, but Quasimodo may be charge nurse during the night shift. *Visit during all shifts* to monitor properly care and staff interaction with the patient on a 24 hour basis. Since the night shift usually begins after visiting hours and ends before visiting hours begin on the following day, you may have to make special arrangements to gain access during this period. It can be done, but not too often.

Arrange to *eat a meal* at the nursing home. Do not expect gourmet food, but check to see if they followed the menu, that the food is warm, adequate and consistent with the patient's dietary restrictions.

Is your patient properly *prepared to eat?*
Are the patient's glasses on and dentures in?
If the patient cannot see, does the staff describe the food location on the patient's plate to her in terms of the face of a clock?
If the patient is impaired, are packages open, meat cut and the dishes appropriate?

WHAT TO LOOK FOR

The most important factor to be observed is the interaction between the staff and the patient. If, for example, the resident is a formal individual, she may resent being addressed by her first name in a condescending manner by a young nursing assistant. A careful watch of the staff as they make their rounds should reveal if there is a trusting and caring relationship.

ITEMS TO CHECK

Are the patient and medical care plans being followed?
Are the necessary therapies scheduled and performed?
If chemical or physical restraints are used, why?
Is the patient's call bell accessible?
Are the roommates getting along?
Is the patient ambulated each day?
How is the resident doing with activities for daily living?
Ask the nurse if the chart reveals any new doctor's orders.
When was the patient last seen by the doctor?

WHEN TO CALL THE DOCTOR

If there has been any significant change in treatment, a doctor should be called. Keep in mind that according to governmental regulations, "Except in a medical emergency, a patient is not to be transferred, discharged, nor is treatment to be radically altered without consultation with the patient or prior notification to the next of kin or sponsor."

If there are new drug orders or the application of restraints, ask the nurse for an explanation. If the reply is not satisfactory, speak with the physician.

BEDSORES (PRESSURE SORES, DECUBITI OR PRESSURE ULCERS)

The surest sign of poor nursing care is bedsores. Except with new admissions or extremely unusual medical conditions which require immobilization, they should not exist. *All pressures ulcers are preventable.* A patient need not be bedridden to develop pressure sores. They are caused by local interference with circulation and usually occur over a bony prominence such as the heel or coccyx. *Check the heels and coccyx* of the resident for the early manifestations of any skin breakdown: a persistently red area and peeling skin.

PROBLEM TIME

GUILT AND MANIPULATION
Maria T., 79

Maria came from a very volatile and emotional family. Two of her six children were adamantly opposed to her entering a nursing home although her doctor recommended it for stabilization of her diabetes and congestive heart failure. She was usually a cheerful and cooperative patient, a condition which changed radically every Sunday morning. On Sundays, which were her family's visiting day, she would awaken early and immediately begin groaning. Her call bell would buzz constantly as she demanded constant service of a frivolous nature. By the time her family arrived she was nearly hysterical, and the staff was disgusted and intolerant of her attitude. This gave Maria ample opportunity to point out to her family how much the nurses hated her, would not help her and ignored her simplest requests.

The situation enraged the family, who also suffered from guilt over the placement. They took Maria's complaints as a rally cry for battle, and fanned out through the nursing home verbally attacking any individual of authority. By the end of visiting hours everyone was exhausted, the nursing staff was disgusted and the administration was considering means to have Maria transferred.

This case clearly illustrates the origination of two types of complaints commonly found in a nursing home: complaints caused by guilt and manipulation. Maria is obviously manipulating her family through her perception of their guilt. They, in turn, are unable to confront the true cause of their feelings, and lash out at a common enemy. This type of frivolous complaining is not only detrimental to the patient's health and adjustment, but will cause the nursing staff to have negative feelings toward Maria as a patient.

AGGRESSIVE COMPLAINTS

An attitude by a resident, family or friends that a strong attack on the staff keeps them on their toes is counterproductive. Nursing home stays can be lengthy, and in order for the relationship between patient and staff to work, it must be composed of mutual respect and caring. Engendering negative attitudes in the nursing personnel can only harm the patient. This is not to say that they will consciously neglect a difficult patient, but it might mean that they will not take that extra step or two which makes the difference between adequate and good care.

TO WHOM TO COMPLAIN

Without question, there will be times when legitimate complaints will be necessary. They should be ranked according to importance. If the patient's safety is in jeopardy, if medical orders are not followed or are improperly executed or if sloppy nursing care has caused such problems as bedsores, you have a very important complaint and should address the problem accordingly.

Many complaints may be minor in nature such as these: Dad isn't shaved today; the housekeeping in the room is poor; or a tissue box is empty. A *positive approach* to the floor staff is recommended for these minor complaints.

Rushing to the nursing station and demanding that dad be shaved immediately or that the floor be mopped at once is not conducive for creating a cooperative attitude. Your statement can be phrased in such a way that will endear you to the staff. You may say that you know they are short–handed that day and you wonder if an electric shaver might help your father's grooming. Perhaps you might ask where the tissues are kept so that you can obtain some. A positive approach such as these deliver a message to the staff that you are a caring visitor who is concerned about the patient's welfare and will go far in correcting minor deficiencies.

FOOD COMPLAINTS

Since food can be very important to any institutional resident, the individual to be approached with questions depends on the exact nature of the complaint. If the food that arrives either at the dining room table or the resident's room is cold, the wrong selection or otherwise improperly served, the complaint should be directed to the charge nurse when aides deliver the food, or to the food service manager where dietary aides deliver the food. For food that is of poor quality, improperly cooked, or inadequately prepared, the food service manager (the cook in a smaller home) is responsible. The selection of the menu is up to the dietician, while the type of diet (soft, salt–free, etc.) should be discussed with the charge nurse.

IMPORTANT COMPLAINTS

When your complaint is of a significant nature, you should speak with the proper supervisory personnel in an ascending order on the chain of command. Give each person opportunity to correct the problem, or satisfy you that appropriate measures will be taken. The first contact should be with the unit's charge nurse, and secondly the director of nursing (perhaps the assistant director if the establishment is quite large). If you still do not have satisfaction, an approach should be made to the assistant administrator or administrator.

At the same time you are making these contacts, you should also be in touch with the patient's doctor concerning the problem. As an attending physician at the facility, the doctor has access to management who in turn will pay attention to his comments.

Since many nursing homes are owned by large corporations or sponsored by nonprofit groups, there is an avenue open for complaints above the local nursing home administrator. An approach can be made to the sponsoring board of the nonprofit organization (church, fraternal or other such type of organization). Contact can also be instituted with corporate management of the nursing home chain. Many of these chains run internal inspection teams who handle such complaints. If a complaint is to be voiced to an authority above the local level it is suggested that a specific name be located and a registered letter be sent directly to that individual.

THE OMBUDSMAN

If you have worked your way through the chain of command with your complaint and it has not been resolved, your final appeal is to your state nursing home ombudsman.

Federal regulations and funding through the Older Americans Act requires that each state establish a nursing home ombudsman. This term, Swedish in origin, is defined by *Webster's Ninth New Collegiate Dictionary* as, "one that investigates reported complaints, reports findings, and helps to achieve equitable settlements." These individuals have the power to enter a nursing home, look at records, talk with staff and patients and otherwise thoroughly investigate the complaint. If necessary, they can call on other state agencies for aid. Your local Area Agency on Aging will have the office location and phone number of the appropriate ombudsman for your nursing home.

Unless you have made a gross error and chosen a nursing home that is past redemption, every effort should be made to resolve complaints before transfer is considered. As previously stated, transfer of the elderly is hazardous and usually contrary to their wishes.

CHAPTER 8

THE VISIT

HOW TO CREATE A REWARDING EXPERIENCE

IT'S FOR THE LONG HAUL

Half of us who reach 65 are going to spend some time in a nursing home, although for the majority the stay will be less than 90 days. A quarter of us who reach 85 will reside permanently in a nursing home, and will live there for an average of two years.

When we are admitted, we typically are going to be a widow, 82 years of age, with two chronic medical conditions. Those of us who age without entering a nursing home are obviously going to be very busy visiting friends and family members who are residents. Our visits will fall into the following broad categories:

The visit with a recuperating patient who is presently undergoing medical stabilization, recuperation or therapy, but who has every prospect of eventually returning home. A visit in this category is basically no different than a routine hospital visit. This type of visit is usually more enjoyable than those at acute care hospitals because of the slower routine and less hectic pace of the typical nursing home.

The visit becomes more difficult when the future of the resident does not include an eventual return to independent living. Due to varying degrees of physical infirmities, these patients are permanent residents.

The visit is further complicated if the permanent resident is confused.

What follows is a consideration of the visit as it pertains to the latter two groups of permanent nursing home residents.

It's Party Time

Nana L., 85

Nana is the matriarch of a large tribe. Her family is now represented by four generations that have not only propagated in large numbers, but have prospered with gusto. By mutual consent, arrived at by resounding voice acclamation, the family has declared each Sunday afternoon to be "Nana's Time." At the appointed hour, three gregarious generations descend on the nursing home in various modes of transport ranging from motorcycles to sedate sedans and vans. Their equipment includes trays of snacks which in amount and variety resemble a hungry Swede's smorgasbord.

Their boisterous arrival is timed like a commando raid to coincide exactly with shift change and nurse's report. Three, and often more, of Nana's senior offsprings hover at the nurse's station where they shout a barrage of good natured, but serious questions. Great grandchildren fight for possession of empty wheelchairs for hallway derby races.

The middle generation spreads food across every available surface in Nana's room. They insistently offer succulent chocolate pastries to the roommate, who being too polite to refuse, nibbles on two which will shortly cause her blood sugar to soar.

It is the family's job to cheer Nana, and they proceed in this task with the same gusto they utilize in their approach to all of life's endeavors. They are an amiable group, and their laughter and enthusiasm soon resounds through the halls.

Nana loves her family dearly, but as she grows older she appreciates them more in smaller clumps. She attempts to escape in her wheelchair, but pursued by gleeful ten–year–olds eager to participate in Nana's new game.

By the end of the visit Nana has developed a marked tremor in her hands and a tic in her right eye. It will take her until Wednesday to recover from the onslaught, at which time the dread of the following Sunday will begin.

Nana's tribe is a perfect example of too much of a good thing. This elderly woman would welcome and anticipate a visit by her marvelous family in smaller numbers. One great grandchild, kept away from wheeled furniture, at a time, would have been a rewarding experience. This over zealous family did not consider the ramifications of their actions toward the staff or other residents. As a consequence, the administration was finally forced to speak with senior members of the family in order to point out the problem. This created the initial seeds of disharmony in an otherwise fine adjustment to nursing home living.

THE DON'TS

1. Do not bring unauthorized food.

   Have a full knowledge of your patient's dietary restrictions and conform to those limitations. Be considerate of other residents in the room and general area. Some patients on dietary restrictions might ''kill'' for a candy bar—but it might just kill the resident! These food limits are not just for diabetics, but also for other conditions such as sodium restricted diets and diets limited because of medications.

2. Do not tip for service.

   It is not necessary to give gratuities to any member of the staff. In a good facility, this would be forbidden.

3. Do not visit during the patient's therapy hours.

   If you wish to observe a therapy session, make arrangements in advance. At times, the therapist may wish to teach a new movement, or feel that the therapy for the day requires such concentration that an observer would be distracting. Most physical and occupational therapists are glad to have visitors under controlled conditions.

4. Do not attempt to have long discussions with the nursing staff during shift change, report or meal time.

5. Do not attempt to visit during activities your patient particularly cares for.

   Such an activity might be a social hour that the patient likes, or perhaps only a favorite soap opera that he hates to miss.

6. Do not be too noisy.

   Nana's family was certainly well intentioned, but they inadvertently created a disruptive visit. Elderly minds are less plastic than younger adults, and too much of a good thing can be not only unsettling, but disturbing. A disruptive visit can do far more harm than no visit.

7. Do not bring frightened children.

   Visits by small children are encouraged and usually welcomed by most nursing home residents. However, some small children are confused and alarmed at the nursing home atmosphere. This fear will be transmitted to the patient in a detrimental manner. In such instances, it is recommended that the child be introduced to the nursing home in a gradual and casual manner, perhaps over a period of several days before meeting with the patient.

8. Do not lie!

   This is probably the most common and most serious visiting fault that we have observed. Do not say you are bringing mother home on Tuesday if you are not going to do it. Do not say that Uncle Al is fine when you buried him last Friday. Do not say that Harry is great when he just went back to the hospital for another drying out session.

The elderly seem to have a totality of life experience that allows them to absorb the truth through osmosis. Your lies will be hollow, and more distressing than the truth. Remember, the elderly have lived through most of life's difficulties. They have seen friends and family become ill and die. They can accept the truth and prefer it.

9. Do not play nurse.

Well meaning family and friends who attempt to transfer an immobile resident, ambulate or perform other nursing functions, can be a real danger to the patient. There are many comfort measures and grooming functions that visitors can perform, but establish these with the staff before undertaking them.

10. Do not over visit.

Establish the length and frequency of your visits according to what is most comfortable for you and the patient. Nursing home residents often develop sensitive internal radar that will sense if your visit is under duress or you are impatient to leave. Conversely, some patients tire easily, and short visits are the most beneficial.

Do

1. Do bring snacks, kids and pets.

Goodies from home (keeping dietary restrictions in mind) are a welcome change from bland institutional food. A visit from the newest great grandchild will bring smiles, while seeing her ancient tabby cat will relieve anxiety over the animal's welfare. If the family pet is a Great Dane or esoteric pet of some kind, a quick check with the administration is suggested.

2. Find the right time.

As the day progresses, the elderly tend to tire, and are often ready for an afternoon nap. For some, a visit after the evening meal is an exhausting event. A mid–morning visit, between the hours of 10: and 11:30, is suggested. At that time the patient is up, groomed and still fresh.

3. Keep a visiting schedule . . . most of the time.

Once a mutually comfortable time and day have been arrived at, keeping to that schedule will add anticipation and dimension to the resident's week. This schedule should be occasionally changed by the patient's prime advocate in order to monitor care during off hours.

4. Spice the visit.

A small gift or memento can add zest to the visit. A bouquet of fresh flowers from your garden, the latest family snapshots, a small news article about a grandchild making the college honor roll, the latest mystery from a favorite author—small, but important spices that will not only provide attractive conversation pieces, but help maintain contact with the outside world.

5. Leave notes.

It is helpful to hang a small cork bulletin board in some easily seen location. This board can hold a calendar which indicates significant dates and recent photos, and provide space for a large note telling when and who the next visitor will be.

6. Send a surrogate if necessary.

The elderly nursing home resident may anticipate a visit for days in advance. Cancellation of the visit, or a no–show, can be a devastating experience. If at all possible, a surrogate visitor should be obtained for a scheduled visit rather than a cancellation.

7. Make each visit a positive experience.

8. Let the staff know you are there.

Even if it requires creating a routine question to ask the charge nurse, make sure the staff knows that you and other members of the family visit with the patient on a regular basis. It is important that the staff realizes that there is a network of caring people who are concerned with the patient's welfare.

9. Try a video visit.

A video cassette recording of a family event such as a birthday, wedding or ordinary get–together, can be beneficial and enjoyable for the resident. It allows her to participate vicariously in significant family affairs. The video cassette can also act as a surrogate visitor, or merely as a means to knit the far–flung family together. It has the further advantage of replay. This feature means that it can be either savored more than once, or else played in short segments for those with a short attention span.

COMMUNICATING

The best approach to communicating with the nursing home resident is one of consistency. Do not change your relationship by virtue of the new environment. If you yelled at each other before the admission, continue to do so. If you read to each other, continue to read. If you arranged flowers together, make sure that you bring flowers and material when you visit. Avoid the temptation to assume full responsibility for the visit. *To follow an overly helpful course inhibits the elderly person's ability to control their surroundings and loosens their autonomy.*

The most difficult visits will be the early ones. The initial adjustment period is a wrenching time for all concerned, and habits established during this period will often prevail during many future months. We have emphasized the importance of a positive approach, particularly during the adjustment period. We recommend that all questions frankly asked by the new resident be honestly answered. If questions arise concerning medical matters, they should be answered, just as honest concerns over happenings on the home front should receive a candid response.

COMMUNICATING WITH THE HEARING IMPAIRED

One in every four people over 65 have a hearing impairment to a greater or lesser degree.

The two most common types of hearing problems are otosclerosis and presbycusis. In otosclerosis there is formation of spongy bone, i.e., a kind of scar tissue in the inner ear, and the normal conduction of sound is diminished. Hearing aids can often help this form of hearing loss by amplifying sound. To understand how a hearing aid works, consider yourself sitting in the back of a large auditorium trying to hear a singer on stage. You hear very few of the words until the singer remembers to turn on the microphone and his voice is amplified. An analogous situation would be true for a hearing impaired individual who listens without a hearing aid, and then with a hearing aid. It is important to ensure that hearing aids are properly fitted and are not bothersome to the patient.

Presbycusis is an age–dependent change in hearing that occurs in old age. The cause is unknown. It differs from otosclerosis in that the loss of hearing results from the decline in the function of the auditory nerve. Hearing aids can help presbycusis, especially if an aid amplifies selected frequencies rather than all sound. Some elderly have a mix of both otosclerosis and presbycusis.

Recent research has demonstrated an association between the degree of hearing loss and severity of cognitive dysfunction in the elderly. In other words, dementia can be made worse by poor hearing. This finding has important ramifications for treating dementia, for hearing loss is common, often not detected and infrequently treated. Aggressive treatment of hearing impairments may possibly improve a demented person's cognitive function. *All* elderly patients need routine hearing evaluations.

The general guidelines that are helpful for communicating with the hearing impaired are as follows:

1. Face the listener. If hearing is severely impaired speak directly into their ear.
2. Speak slowly and distinctly, form words carefully and keep words and sentences short.
3. Diminish outside distractions (other visitors, radios and television sets, etc.).
4. Use facial expressions and gestures to help express meaning.

5. Lower your voice in pitch and tone (high–pitched sounds are more difficult to hear).
6. For those with severe impairment, keep writing materials at hand.

COMMUNICATING WITH THE CONFUSED PATIENT

Martha L., 75

After she was widowed, Martha lived alone for several years. Her only child, Rene, visited her apartment every week. Two years ago, Rene became concerned that her mother was not properly taking care of herself. She noticed that Martha was becoming increasingly forgetful, repeatedly left the stove on, made bizarre purchases and had difficulty in properly expressing herself. Rene moved her mother to her apartment, and as Martha's mental ability continued to deteriorate, arranged for a full medical workup. The geriatric assessment indicated that Martha suffered from senile dementia, Alzheimer's type (SDAT).

Rene attempted to keep her mother at home as long as possible. A few months ago Martha began to display uncharacteristic bursts of temper, became incontinent, fell frequently and did not recognize friends or relatives. Rene, who held a responsible position as a bank vice president, was unable to continue home care and admitted her mother to a nursing home.

Rene hated to visit her mother and became emotionally devastated after each trip to the nursing home. "She hasn't the foggiest idea of who I am," she told the charge nurse. "Some days she thinks I am her mother. On the next visit she's convinced that I'm her sister. When I tell her who I am she yells that she isn't even married. She begs for Gram, and when I tell her that her mother died 20 years ago she gets very upset as if she's hearing the news for the first time. A half hour later she asks the same question, and cries again over her mother. I can't stand seeing her this way! It's not her! That is not my mother. There's nothing there to visit. It's a waste of everyone's time for me to come out here!"

Within the limited intellectual and emotional capacity of the present Martha is the woman she was. Many of her life experiences have been lost, but the basic person is still there as is proven by the repetitive grief she suffers over the loss of her mother. We do not know what transpires within a person afflicted with Alzheimer's disease. We can only observe the patient and note the destruction of recent memories as they digress into earlier stages of their life. Eventually Martha will forget how to perform life's most basic functions: Walking will be lost, and after time, eating. The person is still there, hidden behind a veil of memory, terrified by things not understood, fearful as a small child facing the unknown dark, grasping at tendrils of memory that seem nonsensical to others. It must be a nightmarish time. Without the touch and comforting of others, it will be a lonely time.

It is her mother's fear and her own sense of loss that Rene must learn to confront. With counseling, she began a quiet rapprochement with her mother. The first of the new visits were brief, and consisted of mother and daughter sitting close together. Eventually their hands intertwined. Later there would be an embrace, and finally some laughter over a small and newly discovered pleasure.

Rewards can be found with touch and closeness with even the most severely confused patient. For a child, sibling or spouse, the relationship can enter into a new but smaller dimension.

HINTS FOR VISITING THE CONFUSED PATIENT

1. Try and convey a feeling of *reassurance and security*. Body language is extremely important.
2. *Sit next to the person rather than across from her* as the across position is one of authority and can be perceived as threatening.
3. Be sure she can see and hear you clearly. *Avoid outside distractions and noise.*
4. Unless the patient objects, *touch,* hold hands and embrace.
5. Speak as one adult to another and *without condescension.*
6. *Be calm,* keep your movements smooth, not jerky, and without agitation.
7. Give her *time* to respond.
8. *Do not argue.*
9. *Do tactile things.* Touch pleasant things, smell flowers, walk in the sun.
10. *Always be aware of her limitations.*
    Understand that table manners and other social graces may have been forgotten.
    Understand that what is said is often not what is meant. Many confused patients will repeat the last few words spoken to them. For example, a visitor may say, "Remember that Thanksgiving when dinner was so late that we all became so very hungry?" The patient may respond, "So very hungry."
    Understand that after a certain point attempts at reality orientation are useless. Insisting that today is Thursday, March the third, is meaningless to someone who has lost all concept of time. .

HINTS TO GIVE OTHERS VISITING THE CONFUSED PATIENT

Relatives and friends of the confused nursing home resident will either insist on visiting, or due to the long visiting hours in these establishments, will visit without your knowledge. They may not know of the patient's confused orientation. This lack of knowledge can be upsetting for the resident when she senses the reaction she is creating with these new, and perhaps unknown to her now, visitors.

It is suggested that contact be made with all possible visitors prior to their arrival at the nursing home to go over a few things:

Discuss the patient's mental condition and capabilities. Make sure they understand that this is not a psychotic state, nor is it reversible. Fully inform them of what they may expect to encounter.

Suggest that the visits be short. Suggest simple activities.

Explain to them the information covered in the previous section, "Hints for Visiting the Confused Patient."

Some former friends and even close relatives may not be able emotionally to handle this type of situation and cease to visit. Philosophically understand their motivations and accept this possibility as probably in the patient's best interest.

EMOTIONAL DYNAMICS OF THE VISIT

The emotional baggage carried by a family prior to a nursing home admission is not going to miraculously disappear. The first family visit may be subdued, but the dynamics that existed last week or last year will eventually spring forth with renewed vigor. Some of these feelings will affect the quality and frequency of visits.

Guilt, the most insidious of all emotions, will cause some families to over visit. In others, it will preclude them from ever visiting. Some family members will resist a visit because "they can't stand to see Mom that way." Certain individuals will have other feelings that they can neither articulate nor come to terms with.

The patient, particularly during the initial difficult period of adjustment, may cause difficulties. Some elderly residents make insatiable demands on their families. They expect more visits than can possibly be fulfilled. If they are ignored in this respect, they may accuse relatives of selfishness or lack of love. This type of behavior indicates a strong need to establish or regain emotional control.

New residents may also exhibit clinging behavior which is a manifestation of their fear and anxiety. You are their anchor in the world, and they fear you will leave and never return. In this instance, assurance and more assurance is all the succor you can grant.

Some new residents will find the initial visits upsetting because they act as a reminder of exactly where they are. In this event, perhaps visits should be limited during the initial acclimation period.

The variations of human behavior are so immense that it is even possible that you might find that your patient welcomes the nursing home residency. In some cases, the patient has been exhausted by long emotional battles within the family and is now glad to retire from the fray.

THE HOME VISIT

After the initial period of adjustment, which can only be measured by the reaction of each individual, and if medical considerations do not preclude it, the new resident may eventually be ready for a home or outside trip. It is recommended that the first excursion be short and simple.

Prior to the trip, notify the charge nurse of the departure day and hour. Refamiliarize yourself with the patient's dietary restrictions, and ask if any medications should be taken during the outing. If the patient is fully or partially incontinent, take extra pads. If such a device is in use, understand how and when leg bags are changed. Remember that even in warm weather the elderly get chilly and will desire an extra sweater or jacket.

Several simple prior preparations can make a **meal outing** a more enjoyable experience. A luncheon is preferred over a dinner meal because the patient is more refreshed and less likely to feel fatigue. An advance reservation should be made along with obtaining information concerning wheelchair and rest room accessibility. If the resident is even mildly confused, care should be taken that the menu selection is not overwhelming. The patient should be offered a choice of not more than two entrees, and hard to eat foods such as a thick steak should be avoided.

Assuming that **alcohol** will not adversely react with any medication, one drink or cocktail is adequate. The elderly's poor balance and changed metabolic rate will have reduced their alcoholic tolerance.

Social accidents in a public place will occur, but they are not the end of the world. The people who manage restaurants are professionals. They have served elderly people before and they will again—they have seen it all. In the event of a mishap, the primary objective is to correct the situation with the least embarrassment to the patient.

Short **shopping outings** can be a beneficial experience providing they are not confusing to the nursing home resident. Large department stores or busy discount malls can be threatening and overstimulating. Smaller, specialty shops are recommended, and once again the number of choices presented for selection should be kept to a minimum. For example, if a new robe is to be purchased, the ability to take two home for approval would be preferable over an attempt to select from a rack of two dozen.

Family special events, because of the noise and fatigue factor, can be uncomfortable for many elderly individuals who now live a circumscribed life. Great–granddaughter's wedding reception with 600 guests and music by The Grateful Dead may cost daddy a bundle, but great–grandmother may go bananas in such a setting. In most instances, the elderly would prefer to view the church service and then return to the nursing home rather than suffer through a noisy reception. The same circumstances apply for other large and festive family occasions such as Christmas or Thanksgiving where family jubilation can be excessive. The nursing home recognizes holidays, and most residents would prefer to see small groups of family under less boisterous surroundings.

LESS CAN BE FINE

If an acceptable adjustment has been made by residents to the nursing home, **they** will want to see **their** family and friends in small groups. Rewarding visits can be held with confused patients if the variables of the circumstances are understood, while a new and different dimension is added to the relationship. Outings maintain contact with the world, but they should be managed under carefully controlled conditions.

CHAPTER NINE

TYPICAL GERIATRIC MEDICAL PROBLEMS

ROUTINE CARE IN THE SKILLED NURSING FACILITY

THE FALL

Elizabeth R., 81

Elizabeth was a vigorously independent woman. Before retiring she worked as a social studies teacher at the town middle school. Although she never married, she maintained an active schedule by volunteering at the Presbyterian church, working for the Republican Party and collecting any remotely useful piece of junk stacked on her street for trash pickup. She had always been thought of as eccentric, but as she aged her neighbors saw her interest extend from sidewalk junk to the entire contents of their garbage cans.

It was discovered later, during an examination at the hospital emergency room, that her body was a collection of abrasions and bruises from a series of prior falls. The final fall that prompted this exam occurred when she toppled into an empty garbage can in an alley two doors down from her house. She was imprisoned nearly an hour before sleepy neighbors heard her cries.

She was diagnosed with a fractured hip and underwent a hip replacement. After convalescing at a nursing home, she continued as a resident and was soon wandering from room to room inspecting the contents of waste baskets. She fell again and broke the opposite hip. Within a few days of transfer back to the acute care hospital, she died of pneumonia.

Elizabeth suffered from Alzheimer's disease, but because she appeared independent and was tolerated by her neighbors, her family saw no reason to consider an earlier nursing home placement. Since she was a confused woman over 80 with a history of falls, she was a prime candidate for the serious tumbles she ultimately took. Her feet were probably in poor shape, she continued to prowl in areas filled with slick and slippery surfaces, and when she finally fell, she could not regain her balance. Once she broke her second hip, her rapid death was easily predicted.

This tragic account of Elizabeth's falls is painfully common for the elderly. Each year 25% of those age 70 and 35% of those age 75 will fall! Half of all fallers will do so repeatedly. Women are more likely to be fallers than men until age 75 at which time there is no difference.

WHY DO THEY FALL?

Falls may be the result of a disease which leads to sudden loss of consciousness (syncope). Some of the causes of fainting are heart arrhythmias, seizures, sudden drop in blood pressure when a person stands and other acute events which lead to a marked impairment of consciousness. While this may indicate a progressive disease and require medical attention, the majority of falls do not have a medical explanation. **Most falls** are due to age–related deterioration.

Abnormalities of vision, balance and gait are associated with falling. Changes in vision may be the single most important factor in falling.

The integrity of the bones, joints and other soft tissues of the extremities is important in maintaining an erect posture. Maladies of the foot can be overlooked by many doctors and often dismissed by patients as unimportant. Toenails can be cut and bunions removed, but someone must look in order to identify problems. Often patients are too embarrassed to mention their feet to physicians, and doctors are too preoccupied with other diseases to look. It is in this void that the podiatrist becomes an important member of the elderly's health team. Regular examinations should be made by these specialists.

Medications can contribute to a fall. A diuretic (a drug given for high blood pressure or heart failure) can lead to dehydration and syncope when used by an individual who has restricted fluids due to immobility. Any drug which affects the level of consciousness, such as sedatives, tranquilizers, antidepressants, antipsychotics or antihypertensives, can predispose the elderly to falling. Long–term tranquilizers appear to be extremely risky.

THE COST OF A FALL

The toll a fall takes is primarily psychological. Between 3% and 5% of falls result in a fracture, and another 5% cause bruises, sprains, lacerations or abrasions. Falls by the elderly, unlike younger individuals, may result in a fracture, particularly in the wrist, pelvis, backbone or hip. Osteoporosis, a decrease in the amount of bone, accounts for this predisposition to fractures. One-third of all women over 65 will experience a fracture. Hip fractures exact an even higher price. By 80, one in three women and one in six men will have had a hip fracture. As many as 20% of the frail elderly who experience a hip fracture will die because of it. Long-term nursing home stays are necessary for at least half of the survivors. The risk of a hip fracture appears to be lower in individuals with above average calcium intake; thus, many doctors now recommend that all women take calcium supplements every day.

RISK FACTORS FOR A FALL

Poor vision
Poor hearing
Vitamin B_{12} deficiency
Diabetes
Arthritis
Impaired ambulation
Dementia, especially Alzheimer's type
Foot disorders, calluses, bunions, deformities
Medications
Urinary incontinence
Parkinson's disease
Past stroke with one-sided weakness

Forty percent of elderly fallers are unable to get up without assistance, even if uninjured. This is a frightening experience that can create panic in the elderly. A resultant fear of falling can impose restrictions in activity beyond the scope of the injuries suffered. Many older fallers acknowledge a loss of confidence, independence and mobility as a consequence of their fear of falling.

PREVENTION OF FALLS

Falls should be an anticipated event in the frail elderly's lives. The risk factors peculiar to each individual should be identified and preventive strategies devised to counter each one.

Individuals and their families should address environmental risk factors. A home should be rendered "fall-proof" with the same attention to detail one would employ when "child-proofing."

FIG. 6: RISK OF STROKE BY SEX AND AGE

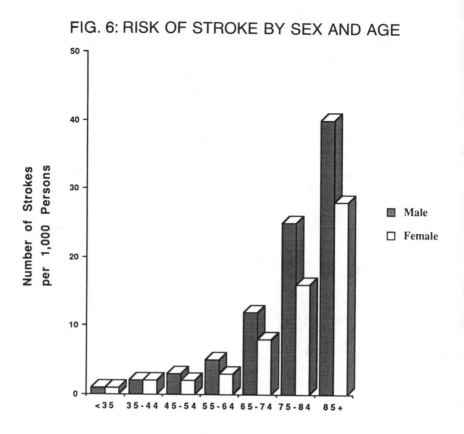

AGE

STROKES
CEREBROVASCULAR ACCIDENTS, BRAIN INFARCTS

Strokes are a major cause of death and nursing home admissions. It is estimated that in the United States 400,000 occur each year. Three–quarters of
all strokes affect individuals between 55 to 85. A third of those stricken do
not survive, but the 5 year survival rate for those that do is a staggering
50%.

Figure 6 demonstrates that elderly men are at the greatest risk of having
a stroke. Indeed, about 40% of all men over 85 will have a stroke.

Stroke victims should have a prompt evaluation of their heart, because
the risk factors for strokes are similar to those for heart disease.

Shirley W., 71

Mutely standing over his wife's bedside, Edward W. wondered how he could have prevented her stroke.

He had always considered his wife a healthy 67–year–old. Although she took daily medication for her hypertension and mild diabetes, the doctor always complimented her after routine checkups for having such good health.

"We should have switched doctors," he thought.

He had found her unconscious on the kitchen floor curled in a fetal position. The faucet dripped into a sink filled with dishes. Water overflowed and formed a puddle around her.

He called, but heard no response. Motionless, he watched the puddle grow. He was convinced that she was dead, and found himself unable to move. He saw her chest move slightly and realized that she was alive. He stumbled to the wall phone and dialed 911.

At the hospital the doctors rapidly established the diagnosis of stroke. A CAT scan showed a large left–sided cerebrovascular accident. They told him that the right side of her body would be weak, and she would be discharged from the hospital to a nursing home in a few days.

Strokes occur suddenly and with a vengeance. The scourge of the combined effects of atherosclerosis, hypertension and an American diet rich in cholesterol and fat culminates in this devastating event. Ischemic strokes occur when a blood clot lodges in a blood vessel and cuts off oxygen to a particular part of the brain. Hemorrhagic strokes occur when blood hemorrhages into the brain tissue.

There are no medical treatments or cures for strokes, only supportive care. Once the medical team at the acute care hospital has determined that the patient is stable, a referral to a long–term care facility will be made. The primary purpose of continuing care is to maintain rehabilitative therapy (rehab), which presumably has already been started.

Rehab does not affect the damage that occurred as a result of the stroke, for this is permanent and irreparable. It aims to improve functions and attempts to restore an individual to an independent and productive life. For unknown reasons the same neurologic damage may cause dramatically different functional deficits in separate individuals.

The most important factors for rehab success are the patients' motivation and their cognitive ability. Motivation may be helped by strong support from the family. If a person has underlying dementia, the expectations for rehab are lowered. Confusion of any sort lowers the goals which are set for any given patient.

Many types of health professionals play important roles during a stroke victim's rehabilitation. The ***physician*** continues caring for chronic medical problems and acts as the team leader, funneling information from the rehab team to the family and patient.

Physical therapists (**PT**) work closely with patients to improve their endurance, strength and mobility. They try to attain independent walking for a previously ambulatory patient, or maintain maximum range of motion in a bedridden person.

Occupational therapists (**OT**) primarily teach skills that are concerned with relearning activities of daily living (ADLs), such as cooking, dressing, grooming, etc.

Speech therapists (**ST**) are trained to identify, assess and rehabilitate persons whose strokes have caused speech problems. In some instances they will work with patients and families to develop nonverbal communication utilizing speech boards, computers, writing, etc. An ST can also make recommendations such as changes in diet for patients with abnormalities of swallowing.

Psychologists are useful in rehab to examine a patient for perceptive and intellectual problems. Because depression can occur in the recovering patient, a psychologist may be valuable for counseling.

Nurses must be alert for some of the complications of the recovery from a stroke. Shoulder pain is caused by overuse during strengthening and range of motion exercises, and can be prevented by having the patient use the strong arm to manipulate the weak arm. Bedridden patients must be turned every two hours to prevent pressure ulcers. A conscientious nurse is constantly alert for redness or irritation of skin, early signs of pressure ulcers.

If patients are able to ambulate, they must! The attending physician in consultation with the physical therapist and nursing staff will determine how often and how long a patient can be ambulated. This program must be carried out for both medical and psychological reasons.

Remember: Ambulation programs are time consuming and can require two staff members and assist devices. It is much easier for the nursing home staff to place a patient in a wheelchair and forget about ambulation. It is the patient advocate's responsibility to ensure that the ambulatory program is performed as ordered.

Incontinence (the involuntary passage of urine) occurs in some stroke patients. Nurses may perform catheterization (placing a narrow tube into the bladder allowing urine to drain), or utilize condom catheters on men or apply diapers. Dietary measures such as a high fiber diet or introducing prune juice may be helpful for patients with severe constipation.

INCONTINENCE

Henrietta P., 76

Henrietta lived a pleasant life with her son and his family until several weeks ago when she began to experience episodes of abdominal pain. The pain seemed to worsen after a meal, so she began taking five or six TUMS for heartburn. She still felt nauseous after a few weeks, and her family convinced her to see her physician, Dr. Thomas.

The doctor carefully examined her abdomen and was impressed with her nausea's relationship to meals. Dr. Thomas discussed the possibility of a "small ulcer" with her, and prescribed cimetidine (a drug that treats ulcer disease). Henrietta took the medication religiously, but to no avail. The pain did not change, and a new problem developed. She began to wet herself during the day and night. Although she could feel when her bladder was full, she could not reach the bathroom in time. Her room began to smell of urine.

Her embarrassed son, prodded by his wife, spoke with Dr. Thomas about the new problem and was informed that his mother had urinary incontinence, for which there was no treatment except wearing adult diapers. The family did not feel that they could assume this additional care burden and they asked Dr. Thomas for nursing home recommendations.

"I'm not ready to leave home," Henrietta told her friends at the Spruce Hill Senior Citizen's Community Center. Her friends convinced her to take her problem to University Hospital for a second opinion.

DR. THOMAS WAS WRONG

The doctor at University Hospital's Incontinence Clinic looked very young, but he had a bouncy enthusiasm that put Henrietta at ease. Before finishing his examination, he performed a rectal exam. The young doctor told her that she had developed severe constipation, which may be responsible for her urinary incontinence. She would need to have several enemas, which could be given at home. Henrietta learned that her urinary incontinence might abate when the constipation was cleared up.

The doctor was right. Her problem was forgotten in a few weeks.

Major breakthroughs in the recognition, understanding and treatment of urinary incontinence have occurred in geriatrics within the last five years. One–third of all cases are transient: Once the underlying cause is discovered and treated, the problem disappears. A rigorous attempt to find this underlying cause should always be made when the problem develops over a short period of time. For instance, fecal impaction, which ailed Henrietta, accounts for

5% to 10% of urinary incontinence and is especially common in confused patients.

COMMON CAUSES OF TRANSIENT INCONTINENCE

Delirium or confusion (as from acute illness)
Infection, especially a urinary tract infection
Atrophic urethritis or vaginitis
Drugs
   Sedatives
   Diuretics
   Antihypertensives
Depression
Decreased mobility
Constipation and fecal impaction

PROBLEMS OF URINARY INCONTINENCE

In the United States almost one million of the institutionalized elderly are affected by urinary incontinence (UI). In 1983 the Surgeon General estimated the economic price of UI at eight billion dollars a year. A nursing home may devote nearly 10% of its budget to the costs of UI. The human price is also staggering since it is associated with falls, fractures, pressure sores, urinary tract infections, depression and social isolation.

The scope of the problem is dramatic. It affects about 10% of elderly individuals living in the community, 35% of elderly patients admitted to acute care hospitals and 50% of nursing home residents. Although most elderly individuals with UI acknowledge major disruptions in their lives, only a minority seek medical attention for it. Unfortunately, when medical advice is sought, many are told that they are experiencing normal aging and that nothing can be done.

ESTABLISHED AND FUNCTIONAL URINARY INCONTINENCE

Two–thirds of all elderly individuals with UI have *established incontinence* which requires long–term therapy. This is an abnormality in the way the bladder empties. There may be a problem with the nerves that tell the bladder to empty, or there may be an obstruction to outflow of urine which causes dribbling, a less powerful stream, etc. Most of the time a physician with geriatrics expertise can determine the type of incontinence, but occasionally will recommend a referral to a urologist for special studies called urodynamics. These studies can often pinpoint the exact problem with bladder emptying, but they are costly, painful and often not readily available.

Some medical centers have incontinence clinics which specialize in diagnosis and therapy of UI. If available, we recommend a referral to one of these clinics, which specialize in the management of this problem.

Functional incontinence occurs as a consequence of non–medical problems. It is common in institutionalized individuals who experience major changes in toilet habits. Nursing home residents are subjected to lack of privacy, lack of control over the interval between toilet use and uncomfortable undergarments. They are more likely to have a debilitating disease that prevents mobility. Similar to transient incontinence, functional incontinence can be helped by addressing issues of privacy, bodily control and mobility.

COMMON TREATMENT STRATEGIES FOR FUNCTIONAL INCONTINENCE

Bedside commode or urinal, if mobility is decreased

Have patient urinate frequently, which decreases amount of residual urine in the bladder

If stress incontinence (i.e., wetting with a cough or a sneeze) do pelvic floor exercises

If there is an obstruction to flow of urine (e.g., cancer or enlarged prostate) undergo surgery to remove obstruction

Consult physician about possible drug therapy

URINARY INCONTINENCE IN THE NURSING HOME

Many families and nursing home staffs consider incontinence an inevitable condition of aging. Unable to cope with this added burden of care, many families consider this the prime reason for nursing home placement. Although a family may have no recourse other than placement, we recommend a complete medical evaluation of UI before this condition is considered the primary reason for nursing home admission.

Far too many nursing homes rely on laxatives, suppositories, enemas and catheters for elimination control of their patients. Control can often be achieved simply by increasing the mental stimulation and social involvement of the resident. Dressing patients in their own clothes may be sufficient to aid in prompting control. In many cases control can be re–established by bladder retraining techniques, which are labor intensive for the nursing staff. Frequently retraining is not attempted, causing the overall condition to deteriorate because of emotionally devastating loss of control, depression and continued social isolation.

A patient advocate should question the medical and nursing staff about the cause and the manner by which UI was diagnosed, and the chosen treatment for it. Is there an incontinence center nearby? Is the patient capable of learning bladder retraining techniques? In the restrained patient, are the restraints still necessary, or are the major tranquilizers still needed? If restraint is required, does the staff respond promptly to the patient's call for assistance? Does the patient with heart failure still need the diuretics? Has retraining been seriously attempted by experienced and knowledgeable personnel? These questions must be answered before allowing the resident's UI condition to become merely a problem of changing clothing and linens.

Many types of disposable incontinence pads are on the market, and each nursing home will have its own preference. These pads should be used judiciously, according to the individual's condition, and not worn all the time. Prolonged exposure of urine to the skin of the frail elderly can cause breakdown and possible pressure sores or infection. In understaffed nursing homes the incontinent patient is at high risk for skin breakdown and pressure sores. Both of these complications of incontinence are avoidable.

The patient's advocate should monitor the nursing staff's attitude, particularly the aides, toward the incontinent resident. It is *intolerable* to berate the patient with such comments as, "Oh, why did you do that?" or, "Why didn't you ring the call bell, you bad girl?" This type of attitude will probably not be apparent while family is present, but by observing the staff care for roommates and others, clues can be overseen and overheard.

Family members should try to understand that aides and nurses are human. That last change of an incontinent patient may be the 20th in a long shift. Staff can become impatient also.

PRESSURE SORES
ARE PREVENTABLE
(DECUBITI, BEDSORES)

Pressure sores are caused by compression of an area of skin between a bony prominence, such as an elbow, heel, shoulder or coccyx (tailbone), and a firm surface. Blood supply to the compressed area of skin is reduced, and if prolonged, the skin will die, break down and form a pressure sore. The elderly patients most likely to develop a pressure sore are poorly nourished, diabetic, bedridden or neurologically impaired. External contributing factors include wrinkling or unevenness of bed clothing or linen, accumulation of sweat and sustained exposure to urine or feces.

Unique aspects of elderly skin also contribute to a predisposition to pressure ulcers. A daily bath is not advisable, for it removes the small amounts of oil that aged skin provides. Dryness from frequent bathing will also cause **bath itch.** Aged skin is easily sheared and requires a long time to heal. Moisturizing lotions should be applied to dry areas for protection. Frequent local bathing may be necessary, particularly if the patient is incontinent.

Prevention is the key word. Patients should not remain in contact with wet sheets or clothing for prolonged periods of time. Bathing should also include gentle drying and the use of lanolin. The single best protection for the nonambulatory is turning (log rolling) by the staff. This frequent change of position should be done at least every two hours.

Using a sheepskin or egg carton pad is also recommended to reduce shearing and increase comfort. Special beds (e.g., Clinitron Beds) are in vogue, but they are an expensive alternative and do not offer any advantage over aggressive nursing. Pads and special beds are helpful, but are not a primary means of preventing sores.

If allowed to worsen, pressure sores can become virtually untreatable. In fact, 60,000 people each year die from complications, usually infections, related to pressure sores. These deaths are preventable!

HEARTS THAT FAIL

Robert M., 72

"I'm tired of hearing you complain about being short of breath. Why don't you do what the doctor says and quit smoking?"

As his wife finished her diatribe, Robert stopped at the top of the stairs leading to the front door and gasped.

Robert was the managing editor of the city's only newspaper and had worked a 10–hour day for the past 45 years. Despite his recurrent bouts of shortness of breath, which his doctor had attributed to congestive heart failure and a previous heart attack, he had not slowed his pace. This week his ankles had swollen, and he had difficulty squeezing into his shoes. Last week he had stopped taking his diuretic because it caused him to urinate too frequently. He had begun using five pillows in order to sleep in an elevated and more comfortable position.

He gripped the porch rail. "I feel like I'm drowning."

Alarmed, his wife stepped toward him, but before she could reach him, he fell unconscious to the landing. Robert was rushed to the hospital and placed in the cardiac care unit. The doctors told him that he had experienced another heart attack, and the congestive heart failure had worsened. He would have to spend time recovering in a nursing home.

Robert's story is a common tale for older Americans. His doctor accurately identified the cause of his shortness of breath as congestive heart failure. This disorder can be a terminal stage of several heart conditions, although coronary artery disease (i.e., hardening and narrowing of the heart's arteries) is probably the most common. The pillows he needed to sleep comfortably and his swollen ankles were clues that his heart failure was worsening.

Heart disease affects more than five million Americans. Interestingly, there has been a steady decline in the mortality associated with coronary artery disease over the past 20 years. Peak mortality was in 1963 in the United States. However, in many other parts of the world, such as in the Soviet Union, Japan and Europe, the rates continue to rise. The reasons for this American achievement remain a mystery, but best guesses include reduced cigarette smoking, decreased consumption of animal fats and better therapy for hypertension.

WHAT PREDISPOSES SOMEONE TO HEART DISEASE

"Atherosclerosis" refers to hardening and relative narrowing of the large arteries. The cause of this disease is unknown. However, several risk factors have been identified: advanced age, high blood cholesterol, high blood pressure, obesity, cigarette smoking and diabetes. As the risk factors increase in a given individual, the likelihood of disease also increases. Aware of these issues, many elderly have countered with lifestyle changes. Exercise, a diet high in fiber and low in animal fat and cholesterol and rigorous control of diabetes and hypertension are all ways to reduce the wrath of heart disease.

FAILING HEARTS AND NURSING HOMES

Two groups of nursing home patients are affected by heart failure: those like Robert who require nursing care focused on the heart problem, and others with heart failure in addition to multiple medical problems. Those in Robert's category are more likely to be discharged from a nursing home after a minimal stay.

The goals of Robert's nursing home admission would be to construct a stable medication regimen, remove supplemental oxygen (if possible) and resume most independent activities of daily living. Through a multi–disciplinary team approach, the goals of this admission can be achieved.

Heart failure may be one of many problems which affect a patient with little hope for resuming independent living. In those cases, in addition to medications, treatment will be directed toward comfort measures. For example, heart failure usually increases a patient's need for supplemental oxygen, which can be the most useful drug the patient receives. If insufficient levels of oxygen are delivered, the patient may initially become irritable and apprehensive. Once a correct amount of oxygen is given, those symptoms rapidly abate.

FROM THE MOUTH TO THE FOOT

MOUTH CARE

Mouth and dental care for the nursing home resident are extremely important whether they are ambulatory or bedridden, confused or not. Poor housekeeping, soiled clothing or uncombed hair are obvious indicators of poor care, but good mouth care is often unnoticed and not performed in the overworked nursing home. This care is of particular importance for the confused patients who are unable to perform basic functions for themselves.

Poor oral hygiene can result in loss of appetite and weight, and be the focus of infection.

For the bedridden patient who is unable to maintain dentures in the mouth, a commercial mouthwash or saline along with glycerin and lemon applied with applicators can be refreshing. This will also cleanse the mouth of food particles.

Nursing homes will have dentists on call who will stop in to check patients. Some facilities will allow a patient's own dentist to call. Most routine care can be delivered bedside, and dental care is often delivered in the beauty parlor because of the seating. Some large nursing homes will have a fully equipped dental office on the premises. Some dentists interested in the care of the elderly have equipped full dental facilities in recreational–type vehicles and are prepared to pull right up to the nursing home to render treatment.

DENTURES

Two of the authors have a young son who, as a part–time dietary aide in a nursing home, managed on his first day on the job to grind up two sets of dentures in the garbage disposal. A thorough investigation into the matter disclosed that one set had been dropped into a cup of coffee, and the other carefully hidden under leftover mashed potatoes. An informal and unscientific study by the same authors reveals that pillow cases are the favored location for hiding dentures.

Rules one through 10 for dentures are *watch out and keep tabs on them.*

Some nursing home residents have dentures which don't fit, and so only utilize them at mealtime. This poor fit can be caused by loss of weight and resulting mouth shrinkage, or swelling of the gums (gingival hyperplasia) due to the body's reaction to certain drugs. Care should be taken to see that dentures and partial plates continue to fit properly as poor fits may discourage eating or cause an abscess.

It is next to impossible to obtain a proper dental mold for new dentures for the extremely confused patient. In this instance, the efficacy of a new plate is nebulous since the very confused patient will be apt to indulge in repetitive chewing without swallowing, and probably should be fed a blended diet.

FEET

Foot care for the bedridden should include sheepskin at the foot of the bed to cut down heel friction, and a footboard or tent to raise the sheet off the feet. If the patient is confined to one position, booties are excellent. Creaming the feet from time to time is also recommended, but prolonged foot soaking only weakens the skin, causes fungal infections and does not appreciably soften the nails. Soaking is discouraged unless it is part of another therapeutic program.

Toenails in the elderly tend to be thick and older people often develop hammer toes. A visit by a podiatrist is recommended on the average of every 60 to 90 days, depending on patient evaluation. This is true for all patients, ambulatory or bedridden.

Patients with diabetes are at high risk for developing foot problems that may require lengthy treatment. Therefore, **no one but a podiatrist or surgeon should treat the feet of a diabetic patient.** Patients should be discouraged from self–care with commercial corn preparations as severe trauma and infection may result.

If foot trouble is due to a circulation or diabetic problem, Medicare will pay for the cost of a podiatrist. For routine foot care the charges will be in the neighborhood of $50 for a first visit and $25 to $35 for follow–up visits.

CHAPTER 10

THE CONFUSED PATIENT

AN EXPLORATION OF DEMENTIA

THE MYTH OF SENILITY

The myth of senility permeates our culture and casts a cloak of alarm over the elderly when they notice mild forgetfulness in themselves.

"She's senile because of hardening of the arteries in her head," our Grandmother would say.

Gram combined the concept of hardening of the arteries (atherosclerosis) and senility because she recognized that both occur in older individuals. Yet, it is unclear that aging is necessarily associated with mental decline, just as atherosclerosis is not usually responsible for states of confusion.

The word *senility* has always been used to describe a host of mental disorders which result in confusion in the aged. The *Unabridged Oxford English Dictionary* offers the following definition for senility: "the mental or physical infirmity due to old age." This is the myth we have created, for there is no mental infirmity due primarily to the fact that an individual has aged. The word senility should only be used as an adjective when describing certain disease processes associated with aging such as senile dementia of the Alzheimer's type.

WHEN FORGETFULNESS IS BENIGN

Julia Y., 88

Julia's fear began to show itself in her daily phone calls to her daughter. "I forgot to feed Heather this morning," she said one day with great alarm.

"Don't worry, Mother. A cat won't starve to death if it misses one meal," her daughter replied.

"You don't understand and aren't listening to me! I forgot to feed my little cat. I am going senile. I am losing my mind and before long, you'll stick me away!"

"Nonsense, Mother. The damn cat is too fat anyway."

"Yesterday I couldn't remember your cousin Margaret's married name. Today I forgot the cat. What next?"

"What are you going to wear to Helen's wedding next week?" her daughter asked in an attempt to change the subject.

"The same gray dress and alligator pumps I wore to her last wedding and will probably wear to her next wedding. That is, if I don't go senile first and become a vegetable."

Julia has a mild form of memory loss which is called **benign forgetfulness.** This term refers to forgetfulness which is common to normal aging. It is characterized by a gradual onset of minor memory loss for unimportant aspects of daily life. Although Julia forgot to feed her cat **one meal,** and could not recall cousin Margaret's married name, important details such as the wedding plans were not forgotten. Moreover, she is preoccupied with her memory deficit. Patients with early– to mid–stage dementia may go to great extremes to hide their forgetfulness from other family members. They will usually deny or ignore their problem. Julia's agitation suggests that her problem is not serious. She should be reassured that an occasional memory lapse is a normal part of aging and not a disease.

WHEN FORGETFULNESS IS MALIGNANT

Herbert N., 86

Herbert's widowed daughter, Natalie, with whom he lived, knew that her father had a problem the day he came down to breakfast without shoes or socks. Her father had owned a fashionable haberdashery store for over 30 years, and had insisted that he and his clerks dress impeccably as an advertisement for the shop. That morning he wore gray slacks, creased to a knife–like edge, a snow white shirt with regimental tie, a navy blue sport coat with a red handkerchief in the breast pocket but no shoes or socks.

She had chuckled at what she initially thought was some sort of joke on his part. At first he had looked puzzled, and then as she pointed to his naked feet, he became concerned, and then agitated.

"Why did you take off my shoes and socks?" he had demanded.

"I didn't," she had replied.

"Why did you do it?"
Her laughter faded. "But I didn't."
Herbert's color changed as his face reddened. His face pinched in anger
as he stood over her. "Where are my things!"

Herbert's response reeks of dementia. His confusion stems from forgetting
to perform an activity which is reflexive for most individuals. People with
age–dependent memory loss forget minor, unimportant details; they would
not forget to dress. People with early dementia will either laugh or become
agitated when they are asked a question they cannot answer. Their responses
are thin veils which do not conceal the central issue: the underlying severe
memory loss.

THE AGING OF THE BRAIN

What changes occur as the brain ages?
   When cognitive functions of elderly people were tested several times over
a period of many years, apparently contradictory data were obtained. Some
people had clear–cut declines in scores, some remained the same and some
even improved. Several attributes were noted to affect the results: degree of
education, social support structure and the extent of chronic disease. Thus,
like many other changes in aging, cognitive loss is significantly affected by
environmental influences, which are modifiable and controllable. In fact, it
is now known that with training reasoning and cognitive performance may
be improved.
   Marked changes of cognition found in elderly individuals are virtually
always due to disease. Alzheimer's dementia, for example, insidiously destroys an elderly person's short–term memory and ultimately daily functioning. This is a disease and not a factor in normal aging. Other forms of
dementia, various states of confusion and different degrees of stroke are
additional abnormal changes of the brain, yet the obvious effects that they
have on a segment of the elderly population negatively bias our perception
of thinking functions in all older individuals.
   Similar to other organ systems, the brain undergoes age–dependent changes.
Most advanced elderly people experience some degree of short–term memory loss. The older brain is less plastic and therefore more affected by environmental insults, which partly explains why the elderly are more prone
than younger individuals to confusional states. They also have more difficulty learning new tasks, and experience a decrease in speed with which
they can process information. Nevertheless, overall intelligence remains un-
tainted by aging. IQ does not change until the eighth decade or later, and

then only slowly. Verbal skills actually improve with age and peak in our 50s or 60s.

THE CONFUSION
ABOUT CONFUSION

Confusion is a symptom. It is a sign of a disease, and a reason for it can always be identified. Mild forms of confusion may pass for normal, but as they become more severe, affected individuals spend more time in unusual behavior. Confused patients tend to sleep more, have difficulty sustaining conversation and respond with abrupt, brief, mechanical answers.

Confusion is recognized by a combination of any of the following features:

1. The patient is awake.
2. The patient is disoriented.
3. The patient has impaired short–term memory.
4. The patient has diminished intellectual capacity.
5. The patient exhibits bizarre and uncharacteristic behavior.

There are many different reasons for a person to appear confused. Some forms of confusion are readily curable, some are treatable and some are terminal. Thus, there should be a thorough search for a cause when confusion is first noticed.

Deciding which medical condition is responsible for the confusion challenges the best gerontologists. The clinical picture can be complicated by the simultaneous occurrence of a combination of conditions in the same individual. For instance, the presence of dementia predisposes a person to depression.

WHEN CONFUSION IS REVERSIBLE

The speed with which the confusion progresses is a crucial piece of information. Most treatable conditions will have a **rapid onset,** whereas dementia, an untreatable form of confusion, generally affects the individual gradually. The following reasons can be the cause of an acute change leading to confusion:

1. **Depression:** Some studies have estimated that about one in three elderly people experience some form of depression during their lives.
2. **Social isolation:** A lack of social intercourse and prolonged loneliness can precipitate bizarre behavior and confusion.

3. **Infection:** Fever alone can be responsible for confusion. In general, confusion which results from fever or infection is called **delirium.** A delirious patient appears drowsy and sick, whereas a demented patient is awake and ready to go. As elderly individuals age, their brains tolerate fever less well. Urinary tract infections and pneumonia can lead to delirium which will often clear up after treatment with antibiotics.

4. **Strokes:** The only sign that a person is experiencing a stroke may be confusion. These individuals are usually identified by concomitant weakness or some other neurologic abnormality.

5. **Diabetes:** If blood sugar drops to low levels (hypoglycemia) a person will become confused. Giving sugar to such a patient causes a complete reversal of the confusion.

6. **Heart failure:** As this condition worsens, a patient's need for oxygen increases. Confusion occurs when someone who needs supplemental oxygen is not receiving adequate amounts.

7. **Drugs:** Many drugs which physicians prescribe can lead to over sedation or confusion in the elderly patient. Some of these medications include narcotics used for pain treatment, antidepressants and antipsychotics used for treatment of psychiatric disorders and sleeping pills. Often these medicines are used at the recommended dose for adults, but elderly people may have side effects at these levels. For this reason, physicians should use the following adage when prescribing medicine for the elderly: Go low and go slow (i.e., use low doses and increase them cautiously and slowly). Thus, before a medication is abandoned, its dosage can be adjusted.

8. **Change of environment:** Moving an elderly person from an acute care hospital to a nursing home, from one nursing home to another or from home to a nursing home can lead to a confusional episode. The move may be considered a life–threatening event by the frail elderly as their social network is shattered or they struggle to assimilate into new and strange surroundings.

Depression
A Common Reversible Form
of Confusion

Roland Y., 80

Roland had lived a full and independent life at his small cottage nestled in the foothills of the Berkshire Mountains. His family worried that he might be lonely, but he always replied that his flowers kept him company. If his flowers did not speak to him, they kept him busy. Roland kept to a strict planting and care schedule that had different flowers blooming from the first days of spring to the first autumn frost. The careful garden plan was painfully and permanently disrupted when he suffered a bad fall.

While in an acute care hospital for orthopedic surgery, Roland became combative, confused and developed paranoid thoughts about his family and the staff. He refused medication, and tore intravenous lines from his arm. He had to be physically restrained. His confusion was such that he mixed up the names of his children, could not recall the fall that brought him to the hospital and even forgot that his wife was dead.

After transfer to a nursing home for stabilization and physical therapy, Roland became uncommunicative and refused to eat. His physician added a secondary diagnosis to his chart that indicated senile dementia.

The use of an antidepressive drug did not help Roland's mental state, and his physical condition continued to deteriorate.

A consult was arranged with a geriatric psychiatrist who changed Roland's drug regime, spent a few hours of directive therapy and finally made recommendations to the attending physician and nursing staff.

Roland was well aware that his fall and surgery were going to limit his physical activities and curtail his beloved gardening. The surgery, recovery room and general hectic atmosphere of the acute care hospital put Roland into a slightly confused state that was complicated by his depression. These two events acting in concert exacerbated his symptoms to the point where he gave every outward sign of the demented patient.

Roland reacted positively to a new drug regime and the increased understanding by the medical staff and his family. He showed a marked improvement.

This case history is a dramatic portrayal of how the older, less plastic mind can suffer environmental insult in an unfamiliar place. This change of environment and his depression over his lack of mobility were enough to cause Roland's confusion, which was reversible.

The individual in our society who is at greatest risk for suicide is a widowed white male older than 65 years (Figure 7). In fact, the elderly have the highest suicide rate of any group in the United States. The rate of depression also increases with age, and it seems likely that major depression is causally linked to suicide in the elderly.

At any given time in the community, 1% to 2% of all elderly will be affected by a major depression. For those living in a nursing home, the figure increases to well above 20%. Depressed mood can affect as many as 20% to 25% of demented patients.

A physician in family practice with a large caseload of older patients recently compared major depression to a depressed mood for us: "Ordinary depression is when you are down in the dumps because your dog was just killed. Major depression is when you can't face life because your dog might be killed."

FIG. 7: U.S. SUICIDE RATES IN 1980

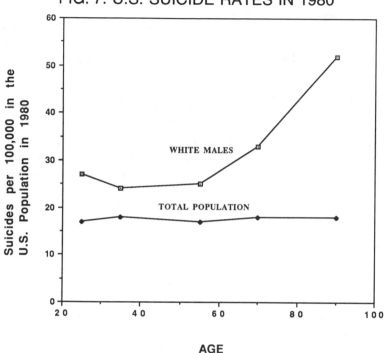

Source: U.S. Mortality Files

Most elderly people handle losses well, since the event usually concerns an anticipated loss. Women usually survive their husbands and recurrently subconsciously rehearse the loss of their spouses. This phenomenon does not occur with men, so a widowed male can be shattered by the unexpected loss of his wife.

SIGNS OF DEPRESSION

loss of interest in life
apathy
social withdrawal
weight loss—very common in depressed elderly
insomnia
fatigue
feeling of worthlessness
guilt
thoughts of death or suicide

difficulty concentrating
memory loss

Because depression may be characterized by memory loss or difficulty concentrating, it may be mistaken for dementia. When a person with depression has severe cognitive impairment (similar to a demented patient), a diagnosis of **pseudodementia** is rendered. As many as 10% of all people initially diagnosed with dementia may really have pseudodementia. The key difference is that pseudodementia is treatable, while dementia is a progressive, terminal disorder. Even depression that occurs in a demented person should be treated, for the individual's social functioning can be improved.

Many common drugs which are prescribed for one of many possible medical conditions can cause depression as a side effect. We recommend that patient advocates understand the nursing home resident's drug regime and associated adverse effects. Simple removal of the offending drug can alleviate the depression.

There are two significant treatment options for depression in the elderly. The class of medication most widely used are the tricyclic anti–depressants. These drugs can be effective in some individuals although the elderly are more likely than younger adults to be resistant to them. The most common side effect of the tricyclics is postural hypotension. Because of this, a person with a history of falls should avoid these drugs. Psychotherapy is as effective as drugs alone, and when the two forms of therapy are combined the total effect is greater than either alone.

IRREVERSIBLE CONFUSION: DEMENTIA

Dementia affects a significant portion of American elderly: 5% of those over age 64 and 20% over the age of 80. As we have emphasized several times, dementia is not a routine part of aging; it is caused by one of several specific diseases. The most common cause of dementia is **senile dementia of the Alzheimer's type (SDAT)**—see Figure 8. **Multi-infarct dementia (MID)**, a condition which results from several small strokes in the brain, is the second most common cause of dementia. The remaining individuals with dementia have a host of other causes (e.g., Parkinson's disease, metabolic disorders, degenerative disorders, etc.). *One–half* of the patients in skilled nursing facilities are affected with dementia, and it is the most common reason for long–term admissions to nursing homes. Despite a wide range of causes, the principles of care are the same for all forms of dementia.

FIG. 8: CAUSES OF DEMENTIA

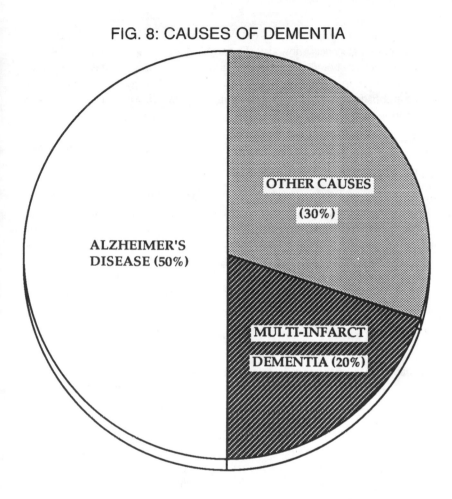

ALZHEIMER'S
DISEASE (50%)

OTHER CAUSES
(30%)

MULTI-INFARCT
DEMENTIA (20%)

ALZHEIMER'S DISEASE

It often seems that each generation of mankind develops a communal fright over some symbolic disease. Centuries ago there was the dread of leprosy. The black death devastated continents during the Middle Ages, quickly followed by small pox. Today, each modern generation trembles before the possibility of a different disease: AIDS and young adults, cancer to the middle-aged, and Alzheimer's for the elderly.

In 1906 at a meeting of the West German Society of Alienists (doctors interested in patients with mental problems), Alois Alzheimer, a 42–year-old neuropathologist, presented his findings. His case concerned a 51–year-old woman who had first experienced memory loss and disorientation, followed by depression, hallucinations, dementia and death, all within five years.

The autopsied brain contained areas of abnormal tissues clumped into what looked like tangled nets (now called neurofibrillary tangles or senile plaques). His audience was bored. No one asked a question. His presentation appeared only as a title in a journal in 1906, and not until a year later was a full report published. Like many important scientific discoveries, Alzheimer's description of a disease, which today is the fourth leading cause of death in the elderly, passed over the heads of his colleagues.

THE HARVARD STUDY

In November of 1989 researchers from Harvard University in Boston published findings that, if confirmed, radically changed the number of persons afflicted with Alzheimer's disease. Their study of 3,623 independently living people in East Boston found that for those over 85 years of age, 47.2% had Alzheimer's.

If their data are corroborated, the projections for total number of people in the U.S. with Alzheimer's would change from 2.5 million to over 4 million individuals!

THE CAUSE

The cause of Alzheimer's disease is unknown. Since the prevalence of the disease has been recognized only in the last 15 years, a great deal of time, money and effort have been devoted to research into its cause. Several hopeful avenues have been encountered, but none have led to an answer. The disease affects individuals throughout the world, and there is no association with nutrition, infections or other environmental factors. A family history can be found in about 25% of the cases, so a genetic predisposition seems likely. All people with Down's syndrome (a genetic condition in which there is an extra copy of chromosome 21) will develop changes in their brain similar to Alzheimer's. Thus, we wonder if the answer lies hidden somewhere within chromosome 21.

DIAGNOSIS

Alzheimer's disease has become a trendy diagnosis in nursing homes. It is a diagnosis of exclusion, which means that other causes of dementia must be ruled out first. A definite diagnosis can only be established at the time of autopsy and an examination of the brain. The difficulty of diagnosis is established by the fact that there is a 15% discrepancy between clinical diagnosis and autopsy findings in cases of adult dementia.

Diagnosis by exclusion can be time consuming and expensive, for several diseases must be investigated. It requires sophisticated tests such as CAT scans and neuropsychiatric testing. All too often the attending physician will scrawl an unconfirmed diagnosis of SDAT (Senile Dementia of the Alzheimer's Type) into a confused nursing home patient's medical record. Given the odds, the diagnosis is probably correct, but since the disease cannot be treated and is irreversible, such a sloppy diagnosis *might* incorrectly label a potentially reversible form of confusion.

SYMPTOMS

Alzheimer's disease progresses through several distinct stages, although timing varies widely. There may be an early or late onset, and a slow or rapid progression. Identical twins, each of whom is affected, may experience quite different forms of the disease. Yet, in all people it is terminal. Survival for more than 10 years after diagnosis is sometimes possible.

In the **early stage** there is memory loss that is difficult to distinguish from benign forgetfulness. You could not pick out an early stage Alzheimer's patient at a cocktail party. At this point, they are affected by generalized memory loss (e.g., forget where things are placed, get lost easily and have difficulty remembering appointments) which may seem related to fatigue or ill health. The early stage is often so nebulous that individuals with strong social skills are able to hide it from their closest friends and family members, although retrospectively it is clearly recognizable.

The mid–phase of the disease is characterized by a progression of symptoms. Forgetfulness increases and long–term memory may be affected. Short–term memory loss becomes more pronounced. Patients may have difficulty in relating to their surroundings. Confusion is now apparent. At some point during the mid–phase, a **realization phase** is entered. Both the patient and family realize that something is wrong. The patient is now at risk for depression. One in four Alzheimer's patients will also have depression.

When memory loss and confusion become so pronounced that the individual cannot function without assistance, the **confusional phase** has been reached. Family members and friends are not recognized. Hallucinations are common. There is a particular hallucination which may be unique to Alzheimer's patients. They perccive the image on the television as real. They may join in conversation with the "TV people," or run screaming out of their room yelling "fire" while watching a newscast of an eight alarm fire. Agitation mounts and immobility and incontinence develop. Eventually all distinguishing characteristics of the person's personality are lost, and the patient becomes **aphasic** (the inability to talk), **apraxic** (the loss of purposeful movement) and **agnosic** (the inability to recognize people or things).

MULTI–INFARCT DEMENTIA

The mental impairment of multi-infarct dementia (MID) occurs as a result of cerebral vascular disease and small strokes throughout the brain. The likelihood of this disease increases with hypertension and diabetes, which are risk factors for strokes. It features a step–like deterioration of thinking functions and an abnormal neurologic examination. These individuals often have abnormal gait and strength in association with their dementia. Its progression is different than Alzheimer's disease in that with each descending step there may be an abrupt worsening, and between episodes there may be mild improvement.

The progression of the disease may be somewhat arrested if the risk factors which predispose the patient to stroke are treated effectively. These factors are similar to those for heart disease: hypertension, diabetes, obesity, high cholesterol, smoking and heart disease. Although this approach is sound, practically it is very difficult to make an impact on the outcome of individuals with MID.

DEDICATED DEMENTIA CARE UNITS

Some skilled nursing homes have created separate units for demented patients. In some areas these are known as dedicated dementia care units. They are also known as Alzheimer's units, confused patient units or other names, such as one we discovered in a skilled nursing home which called itself, "Our Neighborhood." When selecting such a unit, employ the guidelines already mentioned for nursing homes in general, and include the following special criteria:

1. The unit should segregate patients according to level of functioning. Units that mix bedridden terminal patients with those of mid–phase Alzheimer's are defeating their purpose. This does not mean segregation by diagnosis, as functional ability should be the guideline.
2. The dining area should be contained within the unit. There is a wide range of eating habits and abilities among the residents, and they seem to function better in small groups.
3. The unit should be small, numbering between 10 and 20 residents.
4. The staff should be stable in tenure, trained in the limitation and handling of demented patients and sufficient in number to avoid the unnecessary use of restraints. Out of frustration, Alzheimer's patients will often overreact to small failures and become agitated. In this instance, patients should not be isolated, but taken by the staff to a quiet, low stimuli area where they can be calmed.
5. There should be activity programs within the ability of the residents, but none of a childlike nature, and not overactive to the point where the residents will become agitated.

It is quite apparent that these facilities are designed for mid–phase Alzheimer's patients and other forms of dementia where the individual is still ambulatory and retains some cognitive ability. As the disease progresses, transfer will eventually be necessary, but often months or years may elapse.

If these units are run properly, their patients often seem to have a better quality of life than they might at home. Dedicated units are designed to keep confusion and agitation to a minimum, which makes them less frustrating than the constant barrage of the senses that an outside setting would provide.

WARNING

The basic physical plant and nursing standards in a skilled facility approved by Medicare/Medicaid are monitored by state agencies under the mandates of state and federal regulations. However, there are not any special rules for these specialized dementia units. Therefore, unregulated facilities or rest home type institutions will often promote this type of service.

Be careful of statements filled with false promises. It is not possible for an Alzheimer patient to relearn anything! The progression of this condition cannot be slowed or stopped! Any claim for rehabilitative gains in cognitive functions is not only incorrect, but grossly misleading.

AN ENVIRONMENT FOR THE DEMENTED PATIENT

THE PROBLEMS

Maintaining the demented patient at home can be a very difficult undertaking. In addition to the constant surveillance necessary, care increases in difficulty because of the possibility of several common situations:

1. "Sundowning" is a familiar term in a nursing home. It simply means that confused patients sometimes become extremely active at night. At home, when the caretaker is tired and sleepy, this can be devastating.
2. The demented patient will often overreact to minor frustrations (called a catastrophic reaction). These scenes can actually be quite violent and disruptive.
3. Many Alzheimer patients become compulsive "wanderers" in their attempt to leave their home or nursing home. At times, while they are still able, they may even drive cars hundreds of miles in their aimless searching. This type of activity requires constant watchfulness by nursing or home care personnel.

WHAT TO DO

A few essential principles should be followed when establishing a proper environment for a confused patient.

1. Use distraction techniques rather than confrontation during a frustrating situation.
2. The patient's daily routine must be simple and consistent.
3. Personal hygiene and nutrition should be carefully monitored.
4. Each personal possession in a resident's room should have a specific place. Doors and drawers should be labeled with large, easy–to–read signs. Clocks and calendars should be large.
5. Locks or hidden catches need to be placed on certain doors to prevent dangerous wandering.
6. Mildly stimulating activities are fine, but at the first sign of agitation, the activity level should be reduced.
7. The area should be rigorously assessed for unsafe conditions (objects that can be tripped over, etc.).
8. Do not take the word of a confused person such as, "I can take care of myself."
9. A Medic–Alert bracelet or necklace with the patient's name, phone number and the phrase "memory impaired" should be worn.
10. Speak to the patient in a calm, reassuring voice. Speak slowly and distinctly.
11. Never permit a patient to smoke unattended. The home should be assessed for fire hazards.

CHAPTER 11

RESTRAINTS

PHYSICAL AND CHEMICAL

ABUSE

The misuse of physical and chemical restraints is the largest single instance of nursing home abuse.

Every hour of every day over 500,000 elderly Americans in nursing home and acute care hospitals are tied or bound to their beds and chairs. Many of these also nod sleepily like drug addicts on the front stoops of tenements as they are "snowed" by chemical restraints.

This portrait of bound and zonked nursing home residents is the most vivid specter that haunts those who fear these places. It takes little medical knowledge to realize that a restrained patient will shortly become incontinent, and that chaffing by physical bindings against frail skin will often cause bedsores (decubiti). Any quality of life under these circumstances seems virtually nonexistent.

Although the prevalence of restraints in various medical settings ranges from 30% to 86%, and cognitive impairment is also a known risk factor, there has been virtually no research on this subject. There is a prevalent belief that restraints are necessary to safeguard elderly patients, but this has not been clinically proven.

Lee N., 84

Lee was a mustang. As a young high school graduate in the Depression, he had been unable to find work and had enlisted in the army as a private. Commissioned from the ranks at the outbreak of World War II (thus the mustang label), he served as an Infantry Company Commander during the European campaigns. After more than 30 years of military service he retired. Eventually he began to present symptoms that were ultimately diagnosed as Alzheimer's disease. He was admitted to a nursing home as a mid–phase Alzheimer's patient with a diabetic condition that needed stabilization.

The major was a wanderer who often shouted cadence as he marched through the halls and, when he could manage it, out the front door into the street. It was not unusual for him to enter other patients' rooms to "inspect" their bureau drawers. His socially inappropriate remarks and gestures startled other patients and visitors.

The nursing staff felt that he was frightening other patients and placed him in a vest restraint fastened to a wheelchair. The major managed to careen his wheelchair down the halls nearly as rapidly as he could quick march. He was then transferred to a geri–chair (a wheeled chair without self–locomotion). Although he was not able to remove the vest restraint, his arms were free and he became combative toward anyone who came within reach. After his wrists were restrained, he still managed to yell curses and nonsense commands in a voice that carried throughout the building.

Finally, the breakpoint had been reached, and an agitated staff nurse telephoned the attending physician concerning the situation. The doctor prescribed Haldol (a psychoactive drug) as needed. The sedated marching major, now physically and chemically restrained, finally became quiet. He slept a great deal and did not cause the staff further difficulty. He had become a "model patient."

The major also became permanently incontinent and quickly lost his ability to ambulate. He had a marked loss of appetite, and after time developed bizarre facial movements of his jaw, tongue and mouth. He developed terminal pneumonia.

ANALYSIS

We can make several statements that Lee N.'s case history vividly represents:

> After prolonged restraint the continent and ambulatory patient will become incontinent and nonambulatory.
> Restraint of the wandering patient may cause him to become argumentative and combative.
> Since most physicians practice nursing home medicine over the telephone, they will accept a nurse's descriptive account of patient behavior and prescribe medications accordingly.
> Socially inappropriate behavior is not a reason for restraint.
> All too often restraints are ordered for the convenience of the staff.
> Many of the drugs used to treat mood and behavior problems have dangerous side effects. The major's development of odd facial movements is an example of this.

PHYSICAL RESTRAINTS

A physical restraint is an appliance that is designed to inhibit free movement of the individual. It is applied to safeguard the patient against injury, such as falling, or to prevent movement that might interfere with activities of daily living or therapy.

PREVALENCE

In the spring of 1989, a study by the New York State Department of Health reported that 60% of that state's nursing home residents were confined by physical restraints. "Sundowners" (patients who become hyperactive at night) were three times as likely to be restrained as nonsundowners. A late 1970s study found that 85% of residents in Canadian continuous care facilities had restraints in use. Other studies have found that multiple restraints are often the rule, with wrist restraints the most commonly used, followed by chest or jacket restraints, while lap belts are very popular in extended care facilities.

There are several reasons for the variation of results in these studies (although admittedly there are too few studies). Some of the research does not differentiate between acute care hospitals and extended care facilities (nursing homes). Patients recovering from operations, confused or not, and patients receiving life–saving medications intravenously, are often subject to wrist and other types of physical restraints. We are not concerned with the use of restraints in the acute care hospital. What may be medically appropriate in an acute care situation might be completely inappropriate for the long–term nursing home resident.

Some of the studies also include side rails as a type of restraint, and yet often state regulations or medical facility rules require side rail use for patients at night. Many types of side rails can be lowered by the bed's occupant, while others are difficult to lower except by the most agile individual. We are not concerned by the use or misuse of side rails. Hospital beds are high, and nursing home floors are hard. It is the other types of restraints that should concern nursing home residents, their families and advocates.

BASIC PRINCIPLES OF PHYSICAL RESTRAINTS

1. An emergency physical restraint may be applied by a nurse if patients are dangerous to themselves or others.
2. A doctor's order for the restraint must be obtained within 24 hours.

3. The restraint must be removed and reapplied, and the patient monitored for incontinence, toileting and skin breakdown, every two hours.
4. Restraints may not be used for punishment.
5. Alternatives to restraining must be explored before the decision to apply a physical restraint is made.
6. The purpose of the restraint should be carefully explained to the patient, or if that is not practical, to the family.
7. The medical records must document the reason for the restraint.

THE PROPER USE OF PHYSICAL RESTRAINTS

FOR BALANCE

Often stroke patients, those with Parkinson's disease, those subject to seizures or people with certain other medical problems will require body support. They may have one– or two–sided weakness or loss of balance. It is difficult for these residents to sit in any type of chair without either slumping to the side, sliding from the seat or pitching forward. A simple lap restraint (belt) or geri–chair tray will often be sufficient to provide adequate support.

If the weakness is pronounced and affects both sides, a vest restraint may be necessary to keep the patient erect in a chair. At certain stages of their affliction, Alzheimer's patients can become quite rigid and may slide down the chair causing a vest restraint to move up and over their shoulders. There have been documented cases where patients have actually strangled to death under these circumstances. Crotch restraints or T–bars (like in a child's stroller) are used in this situation to keep a patient from sliding. A crotch restraint is difficult to change, and care should be taken with incontinent patients to see that they are diapered and cared for appropriately.

A simple belt or tray restraint can often be removed by patients. It not only provides necessary support, but also acts as a reminder to the patient that their balance is poor, and that they should call for help if they wish to transfer. It is not unusual for a nonconfused patient to have a belt restraint fastened in front.

Raised bed side rails should be sufficient at night for patients who require protection for reasons of balance.

RESTRAINTS FOR MEDICAL TREATMENT

The confused patient who has wound dressings, nasogastric feedings or other treatments that can be disturbed by contamination or flailing may need temporary wrist restraints.

The resident restrained for this reason should be constantly reassessed to see if the confusion or delirium has cleared, or the wound healed, in order that the restraint may be removed as soon as practical.

PUT ON A POSEY

There are a few tradenames that have become synonyms for the product they identify, such as Frigidaire, Kleenex, Scotch Tape, and Xerox. In the medical field, the J.T. Posey Company is associated with physical restraints. "Put on a Posey," is not an unusual verbal order.

The latest Posey catalog shows three generations of Posey women on the front cover demonstrating a Posey lap restraint. The inside page pictures four more Posey family members as the leading corporate officers. The interior of the catalog lists everything from the Posey straitjacket, to "quietly control the most active ambulatory patient" (not used in nursing homes), to the Posey Houdini Security Suit, "for the high risk patient who needs the protection of one of our most secure vests" (occasionally used in nursing homes).

The other items are not nearly so intimidating, and run the full range of physical restraints:

Belts—(safety belts) simple waist supports
Vests—for those who need firm support
Pelvic holders   (crotch restraints) to keep patients from sliding
Limb holders—usually wrist restraints.

These restraints are designed with surfaces that will be the least binding to sensitive skin and give an unusual amount of mobility within their restrictions.

HOW MANY HIPS ARE TOO MANY BROKEN HIPS?

"Patients may be restrained for their own safety."

"Patients with a poor sense of balance, unsteady gait and a history of falls are unsafe to ambulate. Therefore, patients with a history of falls should be restrained."

The statements above seem almost like a syllogism until we consider the ultimate consequence of the conclusion. If a feisty and independent lady who is unsteady on her feet insists on walking, she will eventually fall and may break a hip. Therefore, we shall restrain her in a wheelchair so that she does not fall and break a hip, because a broken hip might not allow her to walk in the future . . . although we know that a restrained patient will eventually lose the ability to walk.

What are we doing?

June T., 90 and Susan M., 69: Roommates in a Nursing Home

Susan had suffered a traumatic head injury which left her susceptible to intermittent seizures. After falling many times at home, she was admitted to the nursing home. June, the older of the roommates, had congestive heart failure and Parkinson's disease, which grossly affected her balance. Neither woman was confused, and they cheerfully got along in their shared room even with the difference in their ages.

Susan was able to self–transfer to her wheelchair, but requested a lap safety belt for protection and as a reminder that she must ring the call bell for aid in walking. The belt was positioned in such a fashion that the Velcro fasteners were at the front, easily accessible to Susan if she so desired. This system worked well, and Susan did not fall during seizure episodes. The only difficulty encountered in this case was when the state investigation team cited the nursing home for restraining Susan without a doctor's order. The doctor's order was overlooked by the staff because they felt that since Susan could release the belt when she desired, that she was not actually restrained.

The same arrangement was offered to June, but she refused. It was obvious that June considered her mobility as her last vestige of independence. The decision was made not to restrain her in any manner except for bed rails at night.

June went down the first time at 3:00 A.M. She had managed to scoot down the length of the bed and slip over the footboard. She took two steps toward the bathroom before stumbling over a side chair and hitting her head on the bureau as she fell. The first fall resulted in a bruise and a few minor lacerations.

Then it seemed that hardly a day went by that June didn't go down. In the hall, by the nurse's station, in the shower—her bruises kept multiplying, but she adamantly refused to ring for aides or use any ambulation device. The falls were charted, the family and attending physician were notified, incident reports were written and June kept falling.

The inevitable happened. The final fall broke her hip.

Everyone involved was convinced that June was aware of the danger in her actions, and her refusal to ring the call bell or accept benign restraints was informed refusal. Some staff members felt that the danger to the patient was so obvious that measures should have been taken without her consent. Others argued that in her particular case, involuntary restraint would have reduced her quality of life so drastically that the benefits were minimal.

If June had been confused, if the doctor had placed an order or if the family had insisted restraints would have been applied. And what was the right answer? We still argue about it.

Interestingly enough, in Canada there has never been a successful lawsuit against an institution for **not using** a restraint. All successful lawsuits have involved the improper application of restraints.

ALTERNATIVES TO PHYSICAL RESTRAINTS

Confused patients who are combative or who are involved in socially inappropriate behavior can be distracted. Staff members should take them to a secluded area where they can be comforted or their interest turned in another direction.

Directed physical activities can be helpful for residents who tend to wander. Guided walking tours for the ambulatory might tire them to the extent that their movement needs are satisfied. Interior units or outside areas can be constructed or altered in such a manner as to be safe for the unsupervised wanderer.

Nursing homes have long visiting hours which means that entrances are open and accessible. There are devices, such as the Wanderguard Monitoring System, that can warn staff when a patient is at an open door. Patients with these Wanderguard protectors wear a wrist alarm similar in size and shape to a watch, but which sets off a beeper at the nurse's station if the patient is within a few feet of an open door.

"Sundowners" can be forced to stay awake during the day to turn around their inner clock.

The important consideration is that a physical restraint should never be applied in the place of proper supervision.

WHAT TO WATCH FOR IN THE PHYSICALLY RESTRAINED PATIENT

In order to monitor your patient in a nursing home, check for the following:

If patients are seated and have a covering over their waists, check under the blanket for the possible presence of a restraint.

If a restraint is properly applied you should be able to slip your fingers under the device.

Check for skin discoloration or pain in the area of the restraint in order to catch possible pressure sores before they become serious.

Ask the charge nurse and attending physician for the specific reasons a restraint was ordered and applied. Remember, *a restraint should never be applied for the convenience of the staff.* Do not accept explanations such as, "we just didn't have the time to watch her," or "he was getting into other patients' rooms."

Make sure the patient seems comfortable and doesn't appear to be constricted to the point of agitation.

Make sure that during waking hours patients are checked every two hours, their position is changed and they are helped to walk or exercise.

Make sure that the use of physical restraints is terminated as soon as possible. Restraint orders written PRN (as necessary) tend never to be re–evaluated.

REMEMBER

Physical restraints have serious side effects. If restrained, the ambulatory, continent patient will quickly become non–ambulatory and incontinent. Physical restraints have even been responsible for several deaths by strangulation. They also cause emotional desolation, cardiac stress and may increase mortality when used for a prolonged period of time.

CHEMICAL RESTRAINTS

Chemical restraints are generally major tranquilizers, sedatives, psychotropic drugs or antihistamines that are given for the specific purpose of inhibiting behavior or movement. These drugs must be prescribed by a physician. The doctor's order, which can be verbal or written, can be designed in one of three ways: as a single dose, as a routine dose (e.g., three times a day, etc.) or as PRN (as needed). Drugs given PRN are distributed by the nursing staff when they feel that the patient requires the medication. Once the doctor writes a PRN order, the nurses need not consult the physician when each additional dose is administered.

PREVALENCE

A study of Tennessee nursing homes found that 42% of the patients were receiving antipsychotic medications, and half of the orders were written PRN. Additional studies have corroborated this and indicated that between 40% and 80% of all individuals in nursing homes are receiving antipsychotic, psychoactive drugs (medicines which affect the cognitive and emotional functions of the mind). As many as half of these patients may receive two or more of these drugs. Most commonly patients or their advocates have not been involved in the decision making process. The drugs have been prescribed without their consent.

Using restraints can be the easy way out for the caretakers of nursing home patients. The most often cited reason for their use is to prevent the patient from interfering with medical care. Simple alternatives can often be substituted for a restraint. For instance, a medication can be given intramuscularly as a shot to a confused "sundowning" patient rather than administering a chemical restraint to prevent the person from pulling out an intravenous catheter. Fever in a terminal patient with dementia could go without treatment, which might obviate the need for a restraint.

CHEMICALS ARE RISKY BUSINESS

The use of major tranquilizers in elderly patients can be risky business. They are most effective in younger individuals with aggressive, delusional or psychotic behavior. When these medications are used in the elderly, confusion, incontinence and disorientation can worsen. In an older person, one dose of a major tranquilizer may have a lingering effect for days. The elderly are also more likely to experience the side effects associated with these drugs.

One standard dose of a major tranquilizer does not affect a sudden outburst of obstructive behavior, a common situation for their use. To produce an adequate chemical restraint, doses large enough to "knock out" the patient are often required. One study, performed in 1960, showed that Thorazine (a major tranquilizer) and a placebo (a sugar pill) had an equal effect in controlling behavior in elderly persons with dementia. Further studies have supported the concept that perceptions of the nursing staff acts as the barometer of a chemical restraint's effectiveness. The frequency with which chemical restraints are used is most closely related to nursing attitudes rather than how well a nursing home is staffed.

To counteract this rampant form of nursing home abuse, the nursing staff should attend educational programs about the appropriate use of restraints. If the attitudes and knowledge level can be changed, then the use of restraints may become less prevalent. Nurses should be taught about sleep disturbances in demented patients, nocturnal wandering, "sundowning," common side effects of major tranquilizers and available alternatives to restraints. They must be taught how to tolerate bothersome behavior without using restraints.

HALDOL: THE WONDER DRUG

Many doctors call this versatile medicine "Vitamin H," a nickname which implies the feeling that a dose a day for all elderly can be a good thing, at least for the medical staff. It can control psychotic behavior. It can transform the meanest lion into a meek mouse. It can restrain the raging bull or the confused wanderer. It is also the most commonly prescribed chemical restraint, accounting for nearly half of all major tranquilizers prescribed in nursing homes.

The *Physician's Desk Reference (PDR)* lists the following accepted uses of Haldol:

1. Management of psychotic disorders (which does not include typical dementia)
2. Control of Tourette's syndrome in children and adults
3. Severe combative, explosive behavioral disturbances in children

Interestingly, the *PDR* makes no reference of its use to restrain confused elderly patients. Most physicians, we suspect, would justify its use by claiming that their patient had organic brain syndrome (i.e., dementia) with psychotic manifestations. Once a physician decides to use a major tranquilizer in order to control the behavior of a patient with dementia, Haldol is generally chosen because of its high potency, relative safety in high dosages and decreased sedative effect, and because generally it causes fewer side effects than other antipsychotics. Some physicians feel that it is especially useful in the confused "sundowning" patient (someone in whom confusion worsens at night). Drugs which have a sedative effect, as is the case with many other major tranquilizers, can actually worsen confusion in a "sundowner" by reducing stimulation that otherwise would maintain his orientation. However, the tradeoff for these advantages is in increased risk of movement disorders, as seen in the case of Lee the Mustang (see the start of chapter 11) during the last days of his life.

Long-term use of major tranquilizers is of unproven and dubious benefit. Nonetheless, any nurse who has given this type of medication for a combative patient will extol its virtues. When confronted with the combative patient, some physicians prefer to use Haldol over other choices because they feel it is more effective under this circumstance.

We believe that long-term administration of Haldol should only be considered with the greatest of care and caution, because restraint is not a recommended use, other options are commonly available and side effects are likely to occur in the elderly, especially women.

TARDIVE DYSKINESIA

Tardive dyskinesia is a dreaded adverse reaction not only for Haldol, but for most of the major tranquilizers that are used in nursing homes. As many as 5% of all elderly individuals receiving these drugs may be affected by tardive dyskinesia. It is sinister for several reasons: Elderly women are the most susceptible, the symptoms are often mistaken or not recognized by the staff and the symptoms may be irreversible. It can occur after a few months of drug usage. As symptoms develop, doctors may mistake them for worsening of the underlying disease. The physician might increase the dose of the antipsychotic medicine and temporarily suppress the symptoms, but tardive dyskinesia returns.

The symptoms of tardive dyskinesia are Parkinsonian tremors (often pill rolling motions with the fingers), difficulty in swallowing and involuntary movements of the face and jaw. There often is continuous, involuntary and abnormal body movements with chewing motions and tongue thrusting.

If these symptoms are recognized in time, the drug can be immediately removed and the condition may not worsen. Failure to recognize and remove the cause will result in an increased severity of these symptoms without hope of reversal.

Other than removing the medication responsible for the tardive dyskinesia, there is no known treatment. Thus, the use of major tranquilizers should be carefully scrutinized and reserved for appropriate indications. The nursing staff should be acutely aware of the early signs of tardive dyskinesia so that the responsible drug can be removed when the initial symptoms appear.

WHAT TO WATCH FOR IN CHEMICAL RESTRAINTS

It has previously been recommended that close contact be maintained with the attending physician concerning the drugs prescribed, the reason for the prescription and possible side effects. This contact is even more important if mood altering drugs are in use. Keep in mind what your doctor would call the baseline, that is, remember what the patient was like before the onset of the drug use, and compare that to what you now observe.

Watch for the following as possible symptoms of overmedication:

Physical Changes

Does the patient seem excessively cold?
Does he complain of dry mouth and skin?
Does the patient have excessive thirst and sweating?
Does he tire easily and sleep a great deal?
Do you observe strange, rhythmic movements of his face, mouth or tongue (tardive dyskinesia)?
Has his walk changed to a staggering shuffle?

Mental Changes

Has the patient become more confused without reason?
Is the patient more depressed and/or agitated?
Has vision changed—staring into space, blurred, etc.?

Watch For

PRN orders (give as needed). Ask that the physician review the need for any medicine ordered PRN every 48 hours.

Investigate the nurses' attitudes toward restraints. If possible, this should be done before admitting the patient to a given nursing home.

CHAPTER 12

DISCHARGE

HOME CARE

IS IT TIME TO GO HOME?

There are several reasons to emphasize home care for the elderly. Patients and their families are motivated by a desire to keep the elderly in their own surroundings rather than the sterile regimentation of a nursing home. Governmental agencies responsible for funding Medicare and Medicaid are interested because the cost is less than half the cost of a skilled nursing home. As a consequence, recent changes in Medicare encourage home care. Several states now screen for potential care levels before they will authorize admission to a nursing home under an entitlement program.

Except for patients whose medical needs require the extended facilities of an acute care hospital, home care is always a possibility—if the family has the ability to pay for the necessary services and expend the physical and emotional tolls it can extract.

A DISCHARGE CHECKLIST

Home care may be appropriate for persons who do not need 24 hour monitoring and skilled nursing. If a patient has progressed to this point, a nursing home discharge could be seriously considered, but certain questions should be addressed:

1. **Is the discharge to be accomplished with medical approval?**
   We suggest that no discharge be considered until the physician feels that the patient is medically stable, the nurses feel that only limited nursing care will be necessary and the physical and occupational therapists feel that some independent living will be feasible.
   We are concerned with those cases where family members, a spouse

or the patient himself brings undue emotional pressure for a return home. A discontented nursing home patient may wish to go home without fully considering the hardships this may cause the care giver. Of particular concern are the frail caring for the frail. We know of examples where a 76–year–old daughter with chronic arthritis attempted to care for her 95–year–old mother, and another where a bedridden 250–pound husband was in the care of his 105–pound, 84–year–old wife.

Obtaining medical approval also assumes that the potential care giver fully understands the patient's medications, medical conditions and needs, treatments and prognosis.

2. **Has a home–care assessment been undertaken?**
   When the patient's advocate is well informed about homemaking requirements, therapy and nursing needs in the home setting, available community services should be investigated. Needs must be compared and carefully matched to what is actually out there.

   Nursing homes are required to have a social worker on staff who can assist in discharge planning. The social worker should be aware of the useful community agencies in your area, their cost and staffing.

3. **Is the primary care giver physically and emotionally able to perform the necessary functions?**
   What we desire to do and what we are capable of doing over a long period of time can be widely divergent. A spouse of 50 years may feel an emotional obligation to take a course of action that is not practical. It is imperative that a premature nursing home discharge not be executed because of guilt feelings or an unrealistic desire for what might be.

4. **Think twice if the patient has a diagnosis of dementia.**
   The patient might have been placed in a nursing home because he had become very confused, wandered in an unsafe manner and was perhaps even combative. As time progresses, some of these symptoms may be ameliorated. The family or care giver may begin to think they can "now handle the situation." Before such a decision is reached, consider the following:

   Remember how difficult the initial nursing home decision was and realize that it will probably have to be made again at a later date if discharge takes place.

   Realize that the patient has progressed to another stage of the illness, and although certain manifestations of the illness might cease, the dementia still exists.

   Around–the–clock nursing needs will increase as patients' awareness of their environment decreases.

5. **Are the accommodations suitable for the patient's return home?**
   If the patient must now use a wheelchair or walker, have ramps been

constructed, rugs removed and a first floor bedroom readied? Have arrangements been made for other medical equipment that might be necessary, such as a hospital bed, a commode, a hoyer lift, oxygen or other such items?

6. **Have provisions been made for continuing medical care and emergency medical treatment?**
   If the patient cannot leave the dwelling, does the attending physician make house calls? Is there a local ambulance service for emergencies? Is wheelchair transportation available?

7. **Have provisions been made for respite care?**
   Respite care is a temporary provision that allows the primary care giver to have some relief. It has been found that continuing care rendered by one individual without "time off" can cause emotional and physical problems that defeat the whole concept of home care. A firm understanding concerning respite time should be established prior to discharge.

8. **Has a reliable health care agency been contacted?**
   If skilled nursing care is required for even part of the day, an established home health care agency should be contacted. This agency should have a case manager complete a home nursing plan prior to the patient's discharge.

9. **What about readmission?**
   If it is probable that the patient will return to a nursing home at some future time, reentry into the same facility would be less traumatic. Has this possibility been considered and discussed with the administration of the present nursing home? This can be an important factor in certain geographic areas with a high occupancy rate in their available nursing home beds.

10. **Is this move for the patient's welfare?**
    Is this discharge what the patient really wants, and can it be accomplished without jeopardizing the resident's physical and emotional safety? Or, is this step being taken because of family guilt feelings?

11. **Is everyone involved in agreement?**
    Are all family members residing in the home in agreement as to the efficacy of the discharge? If mother brings grandma home, but dad and teenage children resent the certain disruption of their lives, unpleasant and even tragic consequences may ensue.

WHERE IS MARY POPPINS WHEN WE NEED HER?

Scanning the newspaper classified ads in our area, we constantly find the following type of advertisement which we reproduce in all its naivete:

"Free room and board in exchange for light housekeeping and care of cheerful, bedridden, senior citizen. Fine home with a loving atmosphere. Extensive references required."

We suspect that the hopeful advertisers expect an aging Mary Poppins to descend miraculously on their doorstep to solve their homecare problems. Needless to say, these ads do not run long, and if they are ever answered, we shudder to consider the possible respondents.

The amazing thing about this optimistic hiring approach is that often the advertisers are somewhat sophisticated people who would not dream of requesting a housekeeper to live in, perform light duties and only be paid in room and board.

Obviously this is not a rational approach to obtain live–in care.

THE COST OF HOME CARE

Zella R., 79

Zella was a patrician New England widow who spent her days managing Highwinds, her large home surrounded by extensive gardens. Her fall might have gone undetected for hours if a zealous gardener trimming the yews hadn't discovered her. She was admitted to an acute care hospital for orthopedic surgery.

Her only child, Lockwood, was an investment banker living in London. He flew home as soon as he was notified of the accident.

Zella's physical recovery was rapid and she was shortly transferred to a nursing home for further recuperation and physical therapy. During his final visits before returning to London, Lockwood became concerned over his mother's apparent short–term memory loss and mild confusion.

Her son took immediate forceful action. He had Zella execute a limited power of attorney, placed adequate funds in the hands of a bank's trust department and left the day–to–day management of all her financial affairs to a trusted local attorney. He hired a registered nurse as case manager and instructed her to obtain a group of licensed individuals for 24 hour staffing. He was able to return to London secure in the knowledge that his mother's welfare was well taken care of.

Zella thrived. Although her confusion persisted, she received nourishing meals and was free to walk the grounds of her beloved Highwinds accompanied by her care givers.

Zella's care was costly. The personnel hired by the case manager were paid at an average rate of $15 an hour, which is $360 a day or $2,520 a week. The base salary rate does not include the employer's portion of the social security, the cost of additional insurance and the management fees paid to the case manager, lawyer and bank. In addition, the expensive overhead of maintaining Highwinds had to be met, along with meals and other allowances to the new personnel.

The total cost to have Zella maintain her life–style was over $200,000 a year. Her son soon calculated that even with his mother's affluent resources, her funds would not last. A nursing home admission was arranged with a part–time nurse's aide as additional help.

In Zella's situation, her case was custodial rather than medical, so licensed personnel were not needed. Homemakers and companions could have been obtained which would have resulted in a savings of about $5 an hour, but the homecare costs of this type of arrangement would still have been extensive.

"Our local home health care agency will provide all the help we need."

Yes, they will, at the following national median cost:

Registered nurse per hour	$26 to $45
Home health aide per hour	$11 to $20*

These agencies have a built–in cost factor from $5 to $7 per hour in order to pay social security taxes, state unemployment charges, insurance fees, training and administration costs and employee benefits, and also include a profit factor.

"We don't have to concern ourselves over cost since Medicare is going to pay the fees."

In all likelihood Medicare will not pay any of the costs. The Medicare regulations are very stringent, but will pay for skilled homecare under very narrow circumstances. See chapter 16 on Medicare and Medicaid for a complete discussion of these benefits.

"Mother only needs someone with her part of the time, so we don't need an agency or licensed personnel. We'll find our own person and save money."

Money can be saved under these circumstances if the right person with at least some training can be found, if the person is known to be trustworthy, if arrangements can be made for backup in the event the primary employee does not arrive and if this individual is able to fulfill your patient's needs.

In years past most communities had a network of individuals who performed these tasks. They had performed these duties long enough to have been at least self–trained, and were usually able to provide extensive lists of local references. Today, most of these people have been attracted to the home health care agencies because of the higher wages, shorter hours and the host of employee benefits available.

---

*Data based on survey by U.S. Select Committee on Aging.

In the event you still wish to contact a freelance individual for these services, we suggest that you call local physicians in family practice, bank trust officers or attorneys active in probate matters for their recommendations of individuals providing these services.

HOME HEALTH CARE AGENCIES

The National Association for Home Care estimates that there are over 5,000 home health care agencies in the country and another 5,000 homemaker agencies. A homemaker can provide light housekeeping, shopping, the preparation of meals, laundry services and companionship. The home health care agencies can provide registered nurses, licensed practical nurses, certified nurse's aides and individuals from the other specialty fields such as occupational and physical therapists.

If skilled nursing care is required, in all but the most complex cases, a licensed practical nurse (LPN) should be adequate. The LPN will cost from $1 to $2 less per hour than the registered nurse (RN). Keep in mind that if medications must be poured, injections given or other invasive nursing tasks performed a licensed person (RN or LPN) will be required. Also remember that in most cases, professional nurses do not perform household chores or laundry not directly related to care of the patient. Separate arrangements must be made for general housekeeping. Aides and homemakers are limited in their functions, but if custodial and personal care is all that is needed, they should be able to fulfill these functions.

Choosing the best possible homecare agency is as complicated as selecting the proper nursing home. In many states these agencies are virtually unlicensed, and even in those states that have some regulations, there are few if any guidelines for aides and homemakers. It is possible that in some areas homemakers might be sent on a case without any training whatsoever.

The National Association for Home Care is a nonprofit professional organization that represents the nation's home health care agencies, hospital home care programs and homemaker health aide organizations. We have abstracted some of the questions they suggest be asked of any home care organization you are investigating:

1. How long has the agency been serving the community?
2. Does the physician know the reputation of the agency?
3. Is it certified by Medicare? (If you cannot obtain Medicare benefits this certification is still a criterion of reliability.)
4. Is the agency licensed by the state?
5. Do they provide a written statement describing services, eligibility requirements and fees?

6. How does the agency choose and train its employees?
7. Does a nurse or therapist conduct an evaluation of needs?
8. Is the care plan written out?
9. What emergency arrangements do they make?
10. Do they insure patient confidentiality?

The primary criteria in your selection of the proper agency is the same as your choice of a physician or nursing home. It is in the individual's training, their empathy toward the elderly and their understanding of the needs of geriatric patients that will ultimately determine their success or failure on the case. If the agency you contact is in actuality an employment agency or nurse's registry, your needs will not be fulfilled unless someone involved is going to act as the case manager.

In order to prepare a list of home care agencies we suggest that you contact your local area on aging, the state Department of Aging, the nearest hospital's discharge planner or a nursing home social worker. You can also contact the National Association for Home Care, 519 C Street, N.E., Stanton Park, Washington, D.C., 20002.

COMMUNITY SERVICES

There is a confusing array of services for the elderly often hidden within the community. Without direction it can be difficult to find an organization or even to realize that a given service is locally available at little or moderate cost. Even with the knowledge that an agency or organization exists, it still might be difficult to locate because of name confusion or because it operates under the umbrella of another organization.

An amendment to the Older Americans Act attempted to rectify this problem by establishing Area Agencies on Aging. There are nearly 700 of these organizations, with locations in every state. They too can be difficult to find since they may be located within another regional agency under another designation. Once found, they will have a great deal of information regarding the availability of services. If you cannot easily locate your Area Agency on Aging, contact your state Department of Aging. This too can sometimes be difficult since the state agency might be called anything from Older Alaskans Commission (Alaska) or Bureau of Maine's Elderly (Maine), to Department of Aging (Illinois and many other states). See the list of state agencies with phone numbers in the appendix.

Another good source of information regarding available services is through members of the clergy. Due to their extensive contact with the elderly, many of the clergy have developed vast and reliable knowledge in this area.

A Short List of Community Services

Adult Day Care or Senior Day Care (Not To Be Confused with Senior Centers)

Adult day care centers are sometimes a part of an acute care hospital complex, a nursing home or a senior center. They provide a variety of services which may include health care, meals, socialization and recreation and often specialized arrangements for demented patients. Some centers have facilities to provide occupational and physical therapy. They not only provide daytime respite for the family, but can act as a halfway house for the recently discharged nursing home patient.

Meals on Wheels

This is a very successful national program funded from a variety of sources with a great deal of volunteer support. In most areas, volunteers will deliver a hot meal each day at noon. A cold meal for later consumption is included in the delivery. Fees are usually on an income–related scale.

Transportation

Some areas have extensive elderly transportation facilities with bus routes from residential neighborhoods to shopping centers and medical offices. Vans with wheelchair accessibility are sometimes available for trips made by appointment. Many congregate housing complexes, retirement villages and life care communities offer transportation service to their residents.

Telephone Programs (Telephone Reassurance Calls)

As a member of a telephone network, the elderly person would receive a daily phone call at a predetermined time. This is not only a safety factor but a chance for socialization.

Respite Care

Time off for the primary care giver is a must! This respite time can be provided by other members of the family or outside arrangements. In areas where there is not a shortage of beds, nursing homes will often provide respite care by allowing for short–term or temporary admissions.

Home health care agencies or nurses' registries will often be able to provide personnel for this service.

Some concerned individuals have formed respite co–ops that trade time back and forth to give each family some relief. If you are going to get involved in a co–op, you must consider the extent of nursing services involved. Most states will allow the immediate family to dispense certain drugs and perform services which would be illegal if rendered by non–family members who are not appropriately licensed.

CHAPTER 13

DEATH

IN THE NURSING HOME
OR HOSPICE

ACCEPTANCE

When I was a young boy in the Oklahoma Territory, there was a night when my father was riding circuit, and the wind blew hard like it does sometimes there. I was afraid to go to bed. My mother held me tight and said, 'don't be afraid of the dark, Billie.' I went to bed then, and I wasn't afraid of the dark.

—the last words of Williams Forrest
to his son Richard

Do not go gentle into that good night,
Old age should burn and rave at close of day;
Rage, rage against the dying of the light.

—Dylan Thomas

The poet Dylan Thomas, unable to articulate his thoughts to his father, projected them in verse. His poem conveys a young adult's feelings of anger and a sense that all one's energy should be expended in the ultimate battle against death.

Elderly nursing home residents have reached a tranquil stage in their life. The words of our fathers and grandfathers suggest that this tranquility is most apt to lead to an acceptance of death in the final days, hours and moments.

Dr. Elisabeth Kubler–Ross interviewed terminal patients and found identifiable patterns in the dying process. In 1969 she published her landmark findings in *On Death and Dying*. The classic sequence of stages of death which she described were denial, anger, bargaining, depression and acceptance. Not all dying patients will experience each stage, and not all patients will follow the typical sequence. Some will get struck in one stage, say depression or anger, and die before finding an acceptance of their death.

155

Anger and depression are often exhibited by nursing home patients, but the underlying causes for these feelings differ from the logical progression described by Kubler–Ross. The frail elderly patient is more likely to be angry over continuing existence rather than death. These individuals are not interested in raging and fighting against death, they are impatiently awaiting their destined appointments. These people are often ready to die because they resent living dependently, are unable to care for themselves and are afflicted by chronic illness.

Many of the advanced elderly have lost their spouse, some have outlived children and all have buried numbers of friends and relatives. They may suffer from more than one chronic condition that is uncomfortable and occasionally even painful. They will often indicate to staff and visitors that they are "ready to go."

We have never seen a patient die in a nursing home troubled with anger or fear. The body seems to sense that it is shutting down and provides emotional protection even for those without medication of any sort. Prior to death these patients enter into a tranquil state characterized by nothing more malignant than an inordinate desire to sleep.

This acceptance of death can also have its dangers. There is a death wish among some elderly that is so strong that they literally will themselves to die. All nursing home personnel are familiar with this phenomenon and call it by many names. It is expressed most simply by the phrase "turning to the wall." These "turned" patients withdraw from all activity so successfully that they can incur acute medical conditions or aggravate existing chronic conditions to the point where they die.

Some patients refuse to eat or allow themselves to be fed. This situation creates a severe ethical dilemma for staff, family and physicians. If patients do not receive nourishment, they will die. The insertion of a feeding tube is an uncomfortable procedure and obviously contrary to the patient's desires. This dilemma is complicated even further by determined patients who rip out the feeding tube, at which time the necessity to restrain the hands physically must be considered.

Nursing Home Deaths

In 1950 half of us died at home. By 1982 65% of us were dying in acute care hospitals and 20% in nursing homes. We can speculate that more people are entering acute care hospitals due to increased medical technology and the advent of Medicare, which would account for the dramatic rise of deaths in our hospitals. The government's newer prospective payment system, with its diagnostic related groups (DRGs), means that more terminally ill patients are discharged to nursing homes. Figure 9 demonstrates an in-

FIG. 9: RATES OF DEATH IN SKILLED AND INTERMEDIATE-CARE LICENSED NURSING HOMES IN ALL 50 STATES

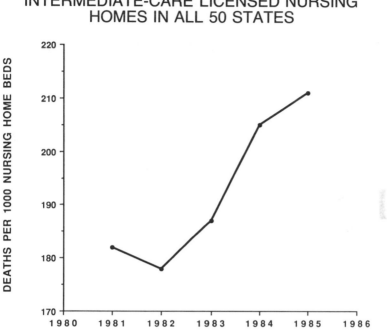

Source: Sager et al., NEJM, 1989

creasing number of deaths in nursing homes following the implementation of DRGs in 1982.

Nursing home patients die from a multitude of causes, but a common scenario is a gradual multi–system failure not specifically attributable to a given diagnoses—in other words, dying from "old age." Death certificates may list the cause of death as heart disease (40%) or pneumonia (29%), but these conditions may be the result of other system failures.

The average age of death for male nursing home patients is 81 years; for female patients, it is 84 years.

PLEASE, NO HEROIC MEASURES

Many elderly fear a vegetative existence where life is maintained by machines. At this point, all thinking functions and most communication avenues have ceased, and only the mechanical performance of these devices allows heart, lungs and brain to register the last vestiges of human life. The avoidance of such a situation is the reason for the creation of the living will.

This document clearly states the patient's preferences toward life sustaining measures. The most important paragraph is as follows:

> ". . . the situation should arise in which there is no reasonable expectation of my recovery from extreme physical or mental disability, I direct that I be allowed to die and not be kept alive by medications, artificial means or heroic measures. I do, however, ask that medications be mercifully administered to me to alleviate suffering even though this may shorten my remaining life."

The existence of a living will, even in those states that do not specifically recognize it by statute, should cause the attending physician to flag the patient's chart with a DNR order (Do Not Resuscitate). Such an order should preclude medical personnel from rushing a crash cart to a patient's room, applying CPR, beginning mechanical ventilation or injecting medicines to restart a heart.

A living will does not prohibit the administration of morphine or other pain killers to a terminally ill patient, even when such administration might slow respiration or other body systems to a dangerous level. It does not discourage the use of comfort measures such as oxygen. The use of oxygen is not a heroic measure, but the use of a ventilator would be so considered. Administering oxygen for individuals with breathing difficulty will make them more comfortable, but will not unnecessarily prolong life.

In most instances, nursing homes are not equipped for the initiation of heroic measures. But, the staff may call the attending physician when a patient is in medical difficulty, and a transfer to an acute care hospital might be arranged. Once the patient has arrived at the emergency room of an acute care hospital, in all probability every life saving measure available would be utilized.

THE CODE TEAM
HEROICS IN THE ACUTE CARE HOSPITAL

Anyone who has spent any time in an acute care hospital is aware of the ubiquitous public address system. What is often not known to the layperson is that each hospital has its own set of broadcast codes. A call for "Doctor Strong to report to the emergency room" is probably a call for security guards to check on an incident in that area. "Call for Doctor Pyro" is a nonalarming signal that there is a fire in the building. Hospitals differ, but the code team call may be a public address request for Code Blue, Team A or Doctor Standstill to report to room so in so Stat (immediately).

Hospitals pride themselves on these teams, and often they can reach a stricken patient in seconds. Each member of the team has a job: Electric paddles are readied, medications are prepared, a breathing tube is inserted

FIG. 10: FINAL OUTCOME OF CPR EFFORTS BY AGE

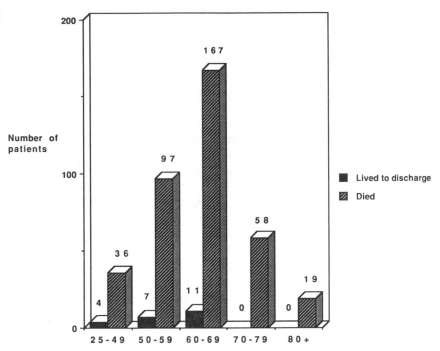

Source: Taffet et al., JAMA, 1988.

into the patient's airway, vital signs are monitored and the rhythm of the heart is closely checked.

Some physicians have called heroic measures for the frail elderly experimental medicine because of the abysmal rate of survival. Taffet et al., studied the outcome of patients who underwent CPR efforts (Figure 10). No patient age 70 or greater lived to be discharged from the acute care hospital! Prompted by these data, some nursing homes have changed their heroic measures policy to require that a doctor write an order if resuscitative measures should be initiated.

Jake T., 78

Jake was a retired school janitor who suffered from congestive heart failure and (COPD) chronic obstructive pulmonary disorder. The congestive heart failure led to pulmonary edema. When he developed pneumonia he was taken by ambulance to an acute care hospital in the next town. Because the COPD had complicated his breathing state, a breathing tube was inserted and he was placed on a mechanical ventilator. His condition gradually improved, and the ventilator was removed. He was sent back to the nursing home for further recuperation and oxygen therapy.

Jake made it perfectly clear to the staff, his doctor and family that he never wanted to undergo a similar experience. His hospital stay had been so traumatizing that he did not want it ever repeated.

Jake's physician discussed this request with members of the family. Everyone agreed, and a DNR order was entered on his chart. The doctor also wrote a note that clearly stated that breathing tubes, mechanical ventilators or CPR were not to be used for this patient.

Jake developed pneumonia a second time and rapidly deteriorated. It became apparent that he would soon die if he was not transferred back to the hospital. Alarmed at their father's condition, the family informed the attending physician that something had to be done.

The doctor explained that Jake was affected by multi–system failures. His heart, lungs and kidneys were all failing.

The family insisted on treatment. The patient was returned by ambulance to the acute care hospital where aggressive treatments were reinstituted.

Jake died in the intensive care unit of the hospital after four days of treatment. He was unconscious for his entire stay, and tubes were in his nose, arms, throat and bladder.

The thread of guilt winds its way through every phase of the nursing home experience starting with the placement decision and ending with death. If Jake's family could have overcome their feelings of past guilt and a fear of potential future guilt because they hadn't done enough, they might have allowed their father the dignified death he desired. If he had recovered from his last acute care stay, his condition would have worsened. His body, unable to tolerate these repeated insults would have been weaker, and he would have been reduced to a near vegetative state.

Living wills, patient requested DNR orders or patient preferences requested in the past are not sufficient to stave off the onslaught of a determined family. If the family demands treatment for mother, grandma or whomever, they will get it! The most compassionate attending physician will bow to this pressure. The legality of living wills in the various states is confusing. Some states recognize their validity, but they can be overridden if the patient is not conscious when decisions must be made. Some states have incorporated the language into legislation as a means to protect the medical community from potential legal liability in the event that they adhere to the request's provisions.

A nursing home resident or potential resident has a measure of protection if a durable power of attorney exists, or some trusted individual is the conservator of the person. If there is only one legal advocate, and the patient cannot speak for himself, the advocate's wishes will be followed.

REFUSAL OF TREATMENT

There is a complicated web of legal and ethical considerations involved in the refusal of medical treatment by a nursing home resident or their family. Legally, an alert and mentally competent individual has the right to refuse any treatment. The "Catch 22" is that elderly patients after the onset of an acute illness are often delirious and confused, and are unable to express their desires concerning treatment. And here's another catch: Medical personnel and family members may also feel that a patient's refusal of treatment is in itself a sign of confusion, and they may act to institute unwanted medical measures.

The answer to this conflict is to firmly establish the patient's desires before the conditions develop. This information should be given to the attending physician and impressed on applicable family members. Then, if patients become unable to discuss these matters rationally during the course of an illness, their advocates can act on the desires as expressed in the past.

Two important studies which underscore the obligation that physicians have to discuss heroic measures with elderly people before illness strikes have been performed. In the first, 75 elderly, healthy members of a senior citizen's club were interviewed. They were specifically asked if they would want to discuss the option of a DNR order with their doctor before they became ill. The group was very willing to discuss their views on death candidly, and 87% said that conversations about DNR should routinely occur.

The second study was in two phases. The physician interviewer asked each patient the following question: "Would you want us to do everything possible to save your life if your heart stopped?" Predictably, the uniform response was, "Yes, of course, Doctor." The interviewer revised his tactics and returned to the patients. He began the second phase by educating each patient about CPR, the intensive care experience, resuscitations and their prognosis for survival after CPR (which he estimated at 3%). Twenty–three of 24 now said that they would want a DNR order. Education appears to be of paramount importance when doctors discuss heroic measures with elderly patients.

Although DNR orders have become common in community hospitals and nursing homes, two–thirds of them are written in the last three days of life when a clouded consciousness might mar the patient's ability to decide. Only 15% of elderly patients are consulted about the DNR order, while 75% of the families make the decision.

The current challenge for health care workers is to address the issue early in the course of a patient's illness.

Ethical Problems

The Debate

Doctors Michael S. Wilkes and Miriam Shuchman in a *New York Times* article on June 4, 1989, entitled, "What Is Too Old?" stated:

> "*Gerontologists maintain that in the treatment of the aged, a kind of intellectual laziness sneaks in when doctors lump every member of this diverse group together . . . Yet, chronologic age so colors the physician's view that the healthy as well as the unhealthy older person is often denied medical options that are presented to others.*"

Medical ethicist, Daniel Callahan, in his 1987 book, *Setting Limits—Medical Goals in an Aging Society,* proposes some principles for limiting treatment of the aged:

> *After a person has lived out a normal life span, medical care should no longer be oriented to resisting death.*
> *Provision of medical care for those who have lived out a natural life span will be limited to the relief of suffering.*
> *The existence of medical technologies capable of extending the lives of the elderly who have lived out a natural life span creates no presumption whatever that the technologies must be used for that purpose.*

This abstract debate becomes quite clear when it is reduced to the consideration of two basic life support systems: the respirator and the feeding tube.

Ethical, medical and legal debates have raged for years over the use of respirators for patients whose conditions were irreversible, or who were existing in a vegetative state. The Roman Catholic Church took the position that a respirator was a machine and thus its use was "extraordinary," which meant that its removal was not killing, but merely letting the fatal conditions run their course. In those states which have various forms of right to die legislation, the plug can be pulled on these machines under certain conditions.

Feeding tubes and forced hydration are another matter. Some states specifically exclude their removal, some legislation is unclear and in other instances there is no case law on the matter at this juncture. Advocates of retaining forced feeding claim that nourishment is a necessity of life and cannot be withheld. This argument avoids the consideration of breathing as a life necessity. The only conclusion that can be drawn is that turning off a respirator usually results in immediate death, while the patient without nourishment may linger for days.

Respirators are seldom seen in nursing homes, so that particular dilemma is avoided. Feeding tubes are another matter as they are often inserted. Any attempt to withdraw a feeding tube will be met by resistance on at least two fronts: by the administration because of their fear of legal liability, and by the nursing staff because of their trained and instinctual need to "hold on" to the patient.

The feeding tube problem is further complicated by patients either with clear mind or in a confused state, who fight the procedure and withdraw the tube. This activity forces the staff and family to approve the use of hand restraints. Some doctors feel that a patient's rejection of a feeding tube, even by the most confused patient, is an expression of treatment refusal, and they will not attempt to reinsert the device as long as the family agrees.

The secret to avoiding the feeding tube problem in a nursing home, with all its attendant complications, is to not have it inserted in the first place. The patient and his advocate should express their feelings to the attending physician before this action is contemplated. The legal problems are not as complex if the device is not inserted in the first place.

THE ANSWER

"What is the Answer?" Alice B. Toklas is said to have asked Gertrude Stein on her death bed.

"What is the question?" was the reply.

Only in the last few years, with the expanding number of elderly in our population, have we begun to ask the right questions. Few of us worry about aggressive medical treatment that utilizes all available technology to save a spry 70– 75– or 80–year–old suffering a first heart attack, cancer or other acute condition. The problems arise at a future time with that same individual as chronic conditions develop and their general health and quality of life deteriorates. When does aggressive treatment stop and pallative measures take over? How long should life be continued and under what circumstances?

The answers lie in a tangle of social, religious, ethical and medical areas. Above all, the answers lie in the desires of the patient, both those that can be expressed in the present, and those values and desires from the past. An objective appraisal and pursuit of those desires is the ultimate gift the patient's advocate can render.

We do not place our loved ones in a nursing home to kill them. They live there because they need that type of care. We have the right to expect that they receive expert and compassionate medical and nursing care. However, it would be less than rational to deny that eventually a point is reached where aggressive measures will not cure, only postpone; will not rehabilitate, only maintain basic life functions; will not dignify, only humiliate; and are not beneficial, but are assuaging family guilt. Within this very personal matrix of judgments and emotions, decisions must be made.

The nursing home resident and advocate must fully discuss with the

attending physician the boundaries of possible treatment *prior to* **any medical crisis!**

These decisions should be communicated to other family members to forgo any possible confrontations at the time of crisis. It must be kept in mind that what is deemed appropriate treatment for crisis number one or two, may be deemed inappropriate at some future time.

THE UNDERSTANDING

The extent of treatment understanding among patient, family and physician should connect with four basic areas of concern:

1. Resuscitation and the do not resuscitate order.
2. Transfer to an acute care hospital with the resulting use of heroic measures such as breathing machines.
3. The treatment of infections with antibiotics.
4. Nutrition and hydration by feeding tubes. Any discussion of feeding as a life sustaining measure includes the use of invasive tubes entering the body, but it does not include feeding aids such as soft diets, a food syringe or other help in feeding.

WHAT DO YOU TELL THE PATIENT?

"Am I going to die?"

This question, when asked by an advanced elderly nursing home resident will be recognized by the nursing staff for what it really means. He is expressing a fear of abandonment, a final need to meet with loved ones, an inner realization that it will soon be time to let go.

The well trained nurse will turn the question around. "Why do you feel that way? Have you spoken to the doctor recently? Would you like to see your family?" Patient and nurse both know that time is limited.

A study of physicians in the early 1960s found that they usually did not tell their terminal patients the true prognosis unless the individual had many economic details to put in order. A similar survey in 1979 found that nearly all doctors told their terminal patients the true facts concerning their medical condition. Many physicians now take the position that when asked, they will always answer the patient's question truthfully.

It is not up to the staff of a nursing home to explain to patients their prognosis. They should suggest that the resident speak with his attending physician.

B.G. Glaser and A.L. Straus in their book, *Time for Dying,* explore four types of awareness concerning death that patients exhibit:

Closed—the dying person does not recognize his impending death even through others.

Suspected—the patient suspects what others know and attempts to confirm or invalidate the feeling.

Mutual pretense—each understand, but pretend they do not.

Open—both are aware and act openly. This permits arrangements to be made and love to be expressed.

This sequence assumes a certain predictability in the illness. However, as is so often the case in a nursing home, the patient may suffer from one or more chronic conditions. Death may occur because of a single condition, or as the result of a multi–system failure. Death may come at any time, or be postponed for months, if not years. There is often no single point where a prediction of death may be made with any accuracy, nor is there any need for such a rigid calendar. At this juncture in their lives, the elderly are aware of their limitations and mortality, and await their judgment either patiently or impatiently.

HOSPICE

Hospice is a philosophy of health care for the terminally ill. The Connecticut Hospice of Branford, Connecticut, the first of its type in North America, states its creed as "To encourage the quality and comfort of existence for the patient and family; and to enhance life for as long as it lasts." They list their goals as:

1. To help patients live out their days as fully and comfortably as possible.
2. To support the family as an integral part of the hospice care.
3. To enable patients to remain at home as long as possible.

The nursing home industry could learn from a visit to the inpatient facility of Connecticut Hospice. The building is light and airy, filled with art work, with nursing stations that do not look like nursing stations. Doors and ramps are not only wide enough for wheelchairs, but are constructed so that beds can be rolled to any part of the building, or outdoors into the gardens or patios. A nursery school for healthy three– and four–year–old children is part of the premises. One hallway has large windows that look into the nursery school classrooms and out onto their playground. This proximity to the young establishes a continuity of existence that words need not express.

It is not a depressing place, and is far more cheerful than many nursing homes. The building and its aura are a testament to what imagination and an innovative approach can create.

This 44–bed facility takes patients for the last several weeks of their life, and operates in close conjunction with an extensive program of outpatient hospice care. The nurse–patient ratio, on a 24 hour–a–day basis, is one to one, and the staff is supported by a large network of volunteers.

There are no life saving machines in a hospice unit. DNR orders do not exist because there are no resuscitations. They do administer oxygen as a comfort measure. A pharmacist makes daily rounds with medical personnel, and as a result they are very successful in controlling pain with drugs taken orally that result in the least possible confusion to the patient.

Seventy–five percent of hospice patients are over 65, and most have terminal cancer. These age and diagnosis categories have recently begun to change as more AIDs patients are admitted into the programs. Hospice patients are aware of their status, and usually have been through extensive acute care hospital therapies. They have now elected to reject further aggressive treatment and die with dignity. Most of the patients have remained at home in the outpatient portion of the program for as long as practical.

The hospice concept is acutely aware of the bereavement problems and stress encountered by families who have a member in a late–stage terminal illness. They have formal bereavement teams that not only counsel families during the patient's illness, but continue to work with them after the death.

A hospice can be a free–standing building, a ward in a hospital or just a concept of treatment for the terminally ill. The first modern hospice was opened in 1968 when Dr. Cicely Saunders of England revitalized this ancient concept with the establishment of St. Christopher's in London. During her travels, Dr. Saunders spoke before doctors and nurses at Yale University in New Haven. It was from this contact that the concept of the Connecticut Hospice was formed. The outpatient program was begun in 1974 and the inpatient facility in 1980.

There are currently more than 2,000 hospice programs operating in the United States and Canada. More than 1,200 of these programs are Medicare approved. The large number of non–approved programs is due to their lack of inpatient facilities. In order to have Medicare approval, a hospice program must have inpatient beds available for its participants. The beds can be in institutions like the Connecticut Hospice or a ward of a general hospital, or the beds can be set aside in a skilled nursing home.

A hospice program may operate through a home care agency, a community hospital, a nursing home or under the umbrella of other health care agencies. It is essential that the program include skilled nursing care, physicians trained in pain control and also homemaker services and bereavement teams that work with the patient and family. The strongest programs have extensive volunteer networks to help in the nonmedical functions.

There are important lessons that the nursing home industry, patients and their advocates can learn from the hospice philosophy.

There is a time when aggressive medical treatment can be refused without an ethical dilemma.

Hospice recognizes the importance of the patient remaining at home as long as possible, and provides the medical, logistical and emotional support to make this feasible.

Hospice programs, through social workers, clergy and volunteers, provide bereavement counseling and aid to the families of deceased patients. This includes, but is not limited to, emotional support, helping with funeral arrangements, insurance collection and other necessary details.

There is a certain predictability among hospice patients. A terminal cancer victim's life span is measurable, while a frail elderly individual with several chronic conditions may die tomorrow or two years from now. However, the lessons are still there to be learned. Would that we heed them.

BEREAVEMENT

If there is any single human emotion that is the most prevalent in the entire nursing home situation from admission through death, it is guilt!

At the death of a loved one, guilt can overwhelm the natural feelings of grief and loss. Guilt over not having done more. Guilt for the things left unsaid. Guilt for the unreasonable anger felt toward the dead . . . anger caused by a sense of futility engendered when the patient lingered on, anger over a sense of abandonment, anger for all the expended effort which now seems fruitless, anger for the bills to pay and the new problems to solve. And then more guilt because of the initial feeling of guilt; this emotion is self–perpetuating.

Guilt must be expunged if the normal channels of bereavement are to be faced and worked through in order that life can return to normal. There is no secret method to suppress this monstrous feeling, but often an awareness of its illogical presence allows it to be partially circumvented.

In a certain sense, death in a nursing home is not as traumatic as in other settings. The patients are older, they have chronic conditions to the extent that death is not unexpected, female patients are usually widows, children of the very elderly aren't so young themselves and death is not usually surprising to the patient himself.

They do not die alone. Geriatric nurses have usually taken care of the average resident for several months. They are not only familiar with the patient and his condition, but they seem to develop a sixth sense concerning impending death. If the family is not present, they will try to contact some member. If the patient is still alone, they will take extra time and diligence to check and be with the patient as much as possible.

CHAPTER 14

LEGAL PREPARATION

THE BASIC STEPS

MAMA WON'T SIGN

Rita T., 84

Rita had always been a docile woman, which was why her present attitude astonished her oldest son, Brett. "She won't sign the damn deed!" He announced in an incredulous voice at a family dinner. "She's agreed to go to the nursing home. She even says she likes the place, but she still won't sign. How in the hell are we going to sell the house on Greene Street if she won't sign? I might point out to everyone that we were going to use that money to pay the nursing home."

"I don't understand it," his sister, Helen, said. "Ma's always been a pussy cat. She never said 'boo' to a goose when Pop was alive."

"She is our mother and not a menagerie," Troy, the youngest son, said. "I don't blame her. She resents being railroaded into that warehouse you two picked out."

Brett threw down his napkin and glowered across the table at his brother. "If you can take care of her, go ahead!"

"Troy has five teenagers at home driving him up the wall," Helen said. "We've discussed this at length. Ma wants to go, and she knows it's best."

"Then why won't she sign the damn papers?"

Rita won't sign because that act signifies something very important to her. It signals the formal end of her independence. Proud men and women, as they advance through the stages of their elderly years, often resent this final loss of control. This resentment and fear can cause resistance to nursing home living, or it can manifest itself in uncooperative acts which are perceived by others as wanton stubbornness.

And yet, it is imperative that certain basic legal steps be taken if an individual is to be admitted to a nursing home. In the case of the frail elderly, or individuals suffering from one or more chronic ailments, the possibility of future mental confusion is present, and its probability must be considered.

TESTAMENTARY CAPACITY

Wills, powers of attorney, trusts and any other legal documents must be prepared and executed while testamentary capacity still exists. Any necessary legal documents should be drawn by an attorney in the patient's state of residence. This lawyer will give specific advice as to the applicable state laws. However, testamentary capacity generally exists if the individual:

understands what a will is,
is able to transact simple business affairs,
has a general knowledge and understands the nature and extent of the
    property involved,
is aware of his relationship to the individuals named in the will and also
    those not named (disinherited).

Living wills must also be drawn and executed while a person is of sound mind. A power of attorney can continue indefinitely during the lifetime of the principle as long as that person is competent and capable of granting a power of attorney, but an ordinary power of attorney lapses with incompetence.

A definition of competence is complicated by the various laws in all 50 states. It is usually obvious to family members when an elderly person has reached a mental state where he might be termed incompetent. Once this stage has been reached, executing any legal document is encumbered by the necessity to establish guardianship. It is far easier to see that the basic legal steps are taken before this situation is reached. Once again, anticipation of future possibilities must be considered.

POWER OF ATTORNEY

Many nursing homes will want to see a copy of an existing power of attorney for a new resident at the time of admission.

A power of attorney allows one person, "the principle," to give to another person, "the–attorney–in–fact," the right to act legally on his or her behalf on limited matters (special power of attorney), or in a wide area (general power of attorney). These legal actions would include banking, paying bills and most other transactions in a person's financial affairs. In most jurisdictions, selling or mortgaging real estate is not included unless the real property is specifically identified in the power of attorney.

In an ordinary power of attorney, if the principle becomes incompetent or dies, the instrument automatically expires.

If a power of attorney is to be utilized for the elderly, it should be a **durable power of attorney.** The laws differ from state to state, but most jurisdictions allow this legal device to survive incompetency.

It is prudent to appoint a "primary agent" for the power of attorney with one or more "successors" in case the primary agent cannot fulfill the obligation. Often, a spouse will be listed as primary agent, but since he may also be elderly and can become ill, an adult child, close friend or even an institution such as a bank, should be named as the successor agent.

Remember to include the ability to make medical decisions! In some states health care decisions can be included in the durable power of attorney, in others a separate living will must be created. Your lawyer will be knowledgeable as to the correct forms to use and the proper procedures to follow.

But We Hold Everything Jointly

"We don't need any of that legal mumbo jumbo because my wife and I have joint checking and savings accounts. Our home title is held as joint tenants with the right of survivorship. That way, if one of us 'goes,' the other gets everything right away without having to wait for probate."

Correct, but? The house and bank accounts may be held jointly, but suppose the nursing home resident becomes incompetent? A joint tenancy requires the signature of both parties on any mortgage or deed. There are certain other assets which cannot be sold or disposed of without both signatures. The durable power of attorney does not change the nature of how your assets are held but it does allow one individual to act in the place of both if the need should arise.

Representative Payee
For Social Security Checks

If a family member has entered a nursing home for other than a relatively short recuperative stay, arrangements should be made to have a representative payee for social security checks. The person designated as the payee will receive and be able to cash the monthly checks. The proper form can be obtained by telephoning the nearest social security office and requesting that it be mailed.

These forms must be signed by the patient and/or his physician. It is an easy procedure, and can be utilized without guardianship or a power of attorney.

GUARDIANSHIP
(CONSERVATOR)

WHAT IS COMPETENCY?

A competent person understands the nature of her actions. She is capable of making decisions that other individuals would make under similar circumstances concerning their own physical well–being and the handling of their financial affairs.

This seems to be a straightforward definition, although each state interprets it differently. There are many areas of argument in trying to define competency. The nursing home resident's advocate is aware of the patient's normal behavior patterns. The advocate will know when the patient's thinking is confused, irrational and inconsistent with logical decision making. The time may come when the individual's actions are harmful to his physical well–being, while financial judgments are jeopardizing the estate. If no prior legal arrangements have been made, it may be necessary to apply to the courts for a *guardianship of the estate* and/or a *guardianship of the person.*

This is a wrenching emotional decision for a family to make since now the court must formally rule on the resident's competency.

APPLICATION FOR GUARDIANSHIP

Application is made to a probate court (called a surrogate court in some jurisdictions). The case is brought before a probate judge for his determination.

A guardian of the estate may or may not be a family member, but is accountable to the court for all financial actions. The guardian (conservator in some areas) has the right to buy, sell or invest any assets that are in the patient's possession. It is assumed that any money spent will be strictly for the patient's welfare, and that the integrity of the estate will be preserved. Under common law, the guardian must make the same sound decisions that any prudent individual would make under similar circumstances.

A **guardian of the person** is granted when individuals are unable (or unwilling) to make responsible decisions concerning their own physical welfare. The guardian can then decide where the incompetent person will live (i.e., a nursing home) and what medical care he will receive, and has complete control over all daily activities.

The mechanics of an incompetency hearing vary slightly from state to state. The alleged incompetent should be notified of the hearing, although it is not necessary that he be present if a doctor submits a report that it would not be medically practical. The person may have legal representation, although it is not always required. The person may present witnesses on his own behalf, although this too is not always required. The court will usually make some sort of investigation, either with their own staff members or by affidavit or interviews with doctors, members of the family and community, and nursing home staff members.

Such proceedings are not uncommon for the advanced elderly. Like marriage, guardianship is a legal condition that is relatively easy to enter, but a great deal more difficult to leave.

Some states will grant a limited guardianship or conservatorship. It is suggested that if any form of guardianship is necessary, that an appropriate attorney be contacted.

ABUSES OF THE SYSTEM

The Cat Lady, 89

We know she had a name, but she will always be known to us as the "Cat Lady." She lived not far away in a small, red, four–room cottage. It all started innocently enough with a pair of kittens who grew into cats and insisted on duplicating themselves several times over. Since the Cat Lady's cottage was near the beach area, the summer resident's abandoned animals soon wandered over. The feline population eventually reached 32.

There was a certain charm in driving by the cottage on a warm, sunny day. Cats curled across the porch roof and they peered out of the overgrown flower beds. Each window had another perched comfortably on the sill.

It was the Cat Lady's grandniece on a vacation trip from California who shrilly complained to the town fathers over the deplorable situation. Not only was the grandniece concerned over the excessive cat population, but she had discovered little human food in the cottage. During her short visit, a man from the light company had arrived to turn off the power. It seemed obvious, she said, that her aunt needed someone to look after her.

An action was brought in the local probate court. The Cat Lady refused to dignify the charges by attending, and was subsequently declared an incompetent. She was placed under the guardianship of a local attorney who promptly arranged for her admission to a nursing home.

We don't know what happened to the cats.

How many cats are too many cats? A full investigation would have revealed that the Cat Lady ate each day through the Meals on Wheels program. She did often neglect to pay her bills, but the utility company was used to this and knew that when their man called he would receive a check. The Cat Lady was eccentric, but she was not incompetent. It is estimated that 400,000 senior citizens are under guardianship.

THE ASSOCIATED PRESS STUDY

In 1987 the Associated Press conducted a year long review of 2,200 guardianship cases throughout the country. They discovered the following:

Almost half of the elderly were not represented by attorneys, and half did not attend their own hearings. One out of four cases had no formal hearing.

A survey by the American Bar Association found that in 25 states advanced age in itself is enough cause to find someone incompetent. Ohio allows the charge of improvidence, while frugal New Englanders in Massachusetts turn thumbs down on a spendthrift. Drunkenness will bring a quick hearing in several states.

Only 14 states require that the elderly be informed of their rights.

Eleven states require no medical evidence, and few states define how doctors should conduct their examinations. Many submitted diagnoses fail to state if the condition is temporary or permanent.

Some elderly discover they are under guardianship after the fact.

Guardians are not always family members. A quarter are friends, lawyers, professional guardians (who get a fee) or governmental agencies.

NURSING HOMES AND GUARDIANSHIPS

A nursing home may request a formal guardianship in order to guarantee payment of their bill. This should be resisted as unnecessary. A durable power of attorney or other legal instrument can assure payment without resorting to an incompetency hearing.

INTER VIVOS TRUSTS
(LIVING TRUSTS)

In addition to any legal and tax benefits that a trust may provide, an inter vivos trust also has strong emotional advantages for the elderly. While mother might still balk at signing over her property or entering into a durable power of attorney, she may be willing to enter into a living trust agreement. In this procedure, she would place the bulk of her assets into a trust created on her own behalf. She would also name a successor trustee (child, spouse, attorney or friend) to take control in the event that she becomes incapacitated. Once again, there are significant legal and tax problems that may evolve in some instances, so a tax accountant and attorney should be consulted.

LIVING WILLS

A living will (see chapter 13) is not a document that should be executed prior to entering a hospital or nursing home; it should be prepared by everyone who has reached their majority (age at which full civil rights are accorded). When we consider the mayhem on the interstate highway system and the general fragility of life, the possibility exists that any of us at any age could be kept physically alive by life support systems without the possibility of future recovery.

And yet, only 9% of Americans have executed a living will to assure that their wishes concerning treatment are followed. The living will has been accepted as ethical by most religions and medical organizations. In a recent survey of physicians, over 78% said they favored withdrawing life support from hopelessly ill or irreversibly comatose patients if they or their family request it.

All fifty states and Washington D.C. have passed laws that give some recognition to living wills. California, Oregon and Idaho have specified the exact legal form of the document, but other states will accept wordage similar to that included in the appendix of this book. Most states require two witnesses who are not family members, and some states require that the form be notarized.

Copies should be given to the attending physician, the nursing home for inclusion in the patient's chart, the patient's attorney and a trusted member of the family or friend.

The living will can be revoked orally at any time.

LEGAL REPRESENTATION

The 1978 amendments to the Older American Act require that every planning and service area, such as the area agency on aging, provide some funds for legal services for low income elderly. No charge may be made for these services, but in some instances a contribution may be suggested.

Lawyers, like physicians, tend to specialize in one or more of the complex fields in their profession. There are attorneys for example, who become experts in probate law or estate planning. This movement has recently been carried one step further when attorney Allen Bogutz founded the National Academy of Elder Law. It is the major goal of this organization to set standards for laws regarding the elderly.

Members of this professional organization are experts who will aid older people seeking help concerning guardianship abuse, equity conversions, pensions, the right to die procedures or other areas of specific interest to the elderly. Nursing home care is particularly complex legally since it involves an interplay between estate planning, governmental benefits like Medicare and Medicaid, guardianships and the right to die questions. Often the ordinary lawyer who may be knowledgeable in probate law may not be aware of the complexities of Medicare and Medicaid benefits.

The names of individual lawyers or law firms who specialize in this field can be obtained from your state or county bar association, or by writing to: National Academy of Elder Law Attorneys, Inc., 1730 East River Rd., Tucson, AZ 85718

PATIENT'S BILL OF RIGHTS
NURSING HOME PATIENT'S RIGHTS AND RESPONSIBILITIES

The Joint Commission of Accreditation for Hospitals has established a set of principles, most of which are now incorporated into regulations for Medicare certified nursing homes. Patients' and their advocates should be familiar with these rights, as it is not unusual for nursing home employees to make statements that are contrary to their provisions. A copy of this statement of rights should be delivered at the time of admission, and a copy should also be prominently displayed in the facility. The major provisions must include:

The right to receive reasonable accommodation of individual needs and preferences.

The right to receive prior notice to change of room or roommate.

The right to prompt efforts by the facility to resolve grievances.

The right for a resident to file a complaint with a state survey agency regarding abuse, neglect or misappropriation of property.

The right to appeal transfer or discharge in accordance with the procedures established by the state.

The right of immediate access by any relative.

The right of reasonable access by others.

The facility must grant to the nursing home ombudsman the right, with a patient's permission, to examine the clinical record.

The facility may not require the resident to waive rights to Medicare or Medicaid or require oral or written assurance that an applicant is not eligible or will not apply for Medicare or Medicaid.

The facility must provide written information on how to apply for Medicare and Medicaid.

The facility cannot require a third party guaranty of the bill.

CHAPTER 15

ALTERNATIVE LIVING ARRANGEMENTS

THE OTHER OPTIONS

INDEPENDENT LIVING

An independent living arrangement for the elderly assumes that residents are not confused, are basically in good health and are able to take complete care of themselves. These are fully functional individuals who are often quite active and vibrant. If they have difficulty ambulating, they use minor assistive devices. They may have, for several reasons, selected a certain type of retirement community that provides at least basic services such as common area maintenance, health and physical security protection and often some homemaking services. The extent of services for life care communities, congregate housing, retirement villages and shared housing are listed in each category in this chapter.

LIFE CARE COMMUNITIES
CONTINUING CARE RESIDENTIAL COMMUNITIES, CONTINUING CARE RETIREMENT CENTERS

Life care communities are an attractive and expanding concept for retirement living. The physical amenities, added to their various levels of guaranteed nursing care, have recently caused a marked increase in construction of these communities. There are two extremely important concepts to keep in mind when investigating such a living arrangement:

1. The required large entry fee is not as safe as sales personnel would lead you to believe. In most instances, payment of this money makes you an unsecured creditor against the development corporation.
2. Do not forget that you are contracting for your future nursing home.

At present there are over 800 life care communities in the United States housing over 250,000 residents.

These communities require applicants to be at least 62 years of age, ambulatory and in generally good health at the time of admission. An extensive financial form, health questionnaire and a substantial entrance fee (often called an endowment fee) at the time of application are required.

Individual accommodations can range from a small studio to luxurious three bedroom apartments or bungalows. The community usually provides one meal a day in the dining room, with other meals available at modest cost. Recreational activities, common rooms, transportation service, emergency medical care and often maid and laundry service are provided at the community. A **skilled nursing home** facility is either on site or located nearby with guaranteed admission for the community residents at no additional cost, or at reduced cost, according to the financial plan of that community.

The units usually have emergency call buttons, cooking facilities and security protection. Residents are asked to eat at least one meal a day in the common dining room as a security check, nutritional protection and as an aid to socialization.

The developers of these projects assume that the prospective residents have sold or are about to sell their mortgage–free homes and will have large amounts of cash available for the entrance or endowment fee. These entrance fees can range from a low of $30,000 to over $200,000. This fee is dependent on the area of the country, the size of the unit, the type of entrance fee refund plan and the amount of pre–paid nursing home coverage. The monthly fees vary in like manner, and can run from a low of $300 a month to over $2,000 a month.

WHAT'S GOOD ABOUT LIFE CARE COMMUNITIES

The properly structured community can provide a high quality of life for independent living for the able resident. If health deteriorates, assisted living or full–time skilled nursing coverage is available. In addition to being able to respond to the resident's health needs with various levels of care, the inclusion of the nursing home in the community means that transfer to that facility does not create a feeling of isolation or sense of abandonment. Entering the nursing home becomes merely another phase of life within the community.

Every aspect of life in these facilities, from the nurse on call to private security police, is designed to create a strong sense of security for the resident. However, it is their guaranteed health care which distinguishes these communities from ordinary congregate living.

Historically, this concept has been extensively utilized by church and fraternal organizations. In the past, these semi–benevolent associations often required the assignment of all assets by the residents in return for guaranteed life care. Private developers, who have recently entered this field, require a large entrance fee, but have also developed plans that return a portion of this payment under certain conditions.

Many communities will refund part of the entrance fee in the event of death or separation from the facility, but will deduct 2% a month of that amount for each month the unit was occupied. This refund would decrease accordingly until it reached a zero balance. Another type of entrance fee plan offers the traditional 2% a month plan or a 90% refundable plan that was payable either to the resident or the estate. Selection of the 90% refundable plan increased the entrance fee by 25%.

There is a wide variation in fees, both entrance and monthly, due to the many types of financial plans offered, nursing care and even the number of prepaid meals a day. Selection of any given plan is dependent upon the individual or couple's financial resources and objectives. It should be kept in mind, as with nursing homes in general, that nonprofit is not cheaper, and that church or benevolent group sponsorship does not mean financial responsibility by that group.

A resident's financial safety, rests with the integrity of the management in their use of the entrance fee funds and their managerial ability. This danger has become apparent to many states, and at the present time 35 states (including Connecticut, New Jersey, New York, Arizona, California, Colorado, Florida, Illinois, Indiana, Maryland, Michigan, Minnesota, Mississippi, Pennsylvania and Oregon), have regulations concerning the establishment of life care communities.

Pitfalls in Paradise: What to Watch for

The new communities we investigated were luxurious and attractive, and had state of the art nursing home facilities. They were also expensive. Entrance fees were in excess of $100,000, and $250,000 was not unusual. The monthly charges would probably exceed most individual social security payments.

Any investigation of such communities should routinely center on the following areas:

1. That the individual units have fire safeguards and call bells in each room including the bathroom. Doors and halls should be wide enough

for the future use of wheelchairs, and carpet piling should be suitable for the use of assistive devices. The placement and height of shelves and appliances should have future years in mind.

2. Outside walks and common areas should have wheelchair ramps, wide halls and appropriate bathrooms.

3. **Investigate the nursing home as if you were going to enter it tomorrow morning.** Utilize the tools suggested in this book to assess the facility. In a new or proposed community, determining the quality of the nursing home can be a problem simply because they are not presently caring for patients, and several important checks are not available. In this instance, obtain the name of the proposed medical director and talk with this doctor in an attempt to obtain his background in geriatrics and understand the plans for this facility.

   Find out how the nursing home beds are allocated. In a typical community of 200 residential units and a 30 bed nursing home, only a few of the nursing home beds might be occupied at any given time by residents. The nursing home would have to admit non–resident patients for economic reasons. In a typical situation of this nature beds should be kept open for their residents at all times. Do they fail to do this?

   Since nursing home stays can extend from a few days to many months, the agreement should be specific in not limiting this coverage. There should be a clear understanding of exactly what happens if nursing home beds are not available when needed.

4. Determine the exact procedure for admission to the nursing home. It is cheaper for the community to care for a patient in a unit rather than the nursing facility. Therefore, management often determines who enters the facility and when. The medical order to enter the nursing home must rest **with your physician.** This provision should be spelled out in the entrance contract.

5. What about nursing care in your home? If medically necessary, is skilled nursing coverage available in your unit for a given number of hours a day over an extended period? Is this cost included in the package? Are there provisions for homemaker and nonskilled nursing care coverage at home? Or do they expect you to hire outside help at your expense? Investigating this aspect of a life care community is important because of the dramatic amount of elderly over 85 who require assisted living (Figure 11).

6. The complete **entrance contract should be reviewed by your attorney.** These contracts are complex. Other questions should be considered, such as what if one spouse dies or a remarriage occurs? What happens if you have financial setbacks and are unable to pay the monthly charges? There are a host of other legal and financial areas that should be investigated and analyzed by your attorney and accountant.

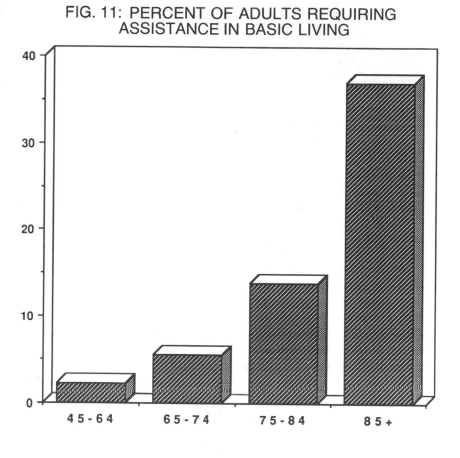

FIG. 11: PERCENT OF ADULTS REQUIRING
ASSISTANCE IN BASIC LIVING

AGE IN YEARS

Your accountant should try to determine if the community has kept,
or will keep, proper reserve accounts for capital improvement, increased health care costs as residents mature, and contingencies for the
unforeseen, such as double–digit inflation or a resident's loss of income.

7. Keep in mind that the monthly charges will rise each year. You must
build into your financial considerations what these charges might be
several years in the future.

THE BIGGEST PROBLEM

Because of fraud or mismanagement some life care communities have gone
bankrupt. Remember, *you have no recordable real estate interest.* Your

contract is an occupancy license that runs to the corporation or the community itself. In the event of a bankruptcy, you are only one of a long line of creditors. You do not have a first lien on real estate or assets, but are an unsecured creditor.

One of the most famous cases of this type of bankruptcy was the Pacific Homes Life Care Community, which had a vague affiliation with the Methodist Church. This community had existed for over 25 years in California (a regulated state) when it went belly–up, leaving all its residents homeless, and some penniless. In this instance, the trustees in bankruptcy reported that the failure was due to years of inept management. It would seem that the reputation of the sponsoring group, the length of time a community has existed or state regulations are not foolproof safeguards.

State regulations do not provide the protection that developers would like you to believe. Some state agencies claim that they are not "regulators" but are actually "monitors" of these communities. In the event they discovered a problem, they would refer the matter to the state attorney general's office for prosecution. This type of procedure could take months if not years before financial mishandling was corrected.

Remember that more than half of the states do not have *any* regulation for these communities except for the nursing home inspections. An overview of those states that do regulate indicates that they usually require financial reserves equal to one month's operating expenses and one year's debt service. These reserves are so thin that a community could be past the brink of disaster before its conditions were revealed.

A community that utilizes present entrance fees to complete initial construction costs or uses these funds to keep down monthly charges artificially in order to attract new residents is operating on the brink of disaster. These projects will eventually deplete their source of fresh funds and will either face a huge upward adjustment of their monthly charges or bankruptcy. Another signal of financial distress is advertising campaigns that suggest you pay an entrance fee now and move in later in order to take advantage of a lower rate. In these instances, the community is probably utilizing present funds for day–to–day operating expenses. To be actuarially sound, new residents should be in moderately good health at the time of their admission. A community that admits new members who are obviously frail and who will shortly need skilled nursing care is in peril. Admitting ill residents destroys the financial concept of these communities and will eventually destroy their financial integrity.

Life care communities can be one of the most attractive and secure answers for elderly housing, but protection of the entrance fee and the complexity of the initial agreement are matters to be investigated carefully. **Caveat emptor!**

CONGREGATE HOUSING
ASSISTED RESIDENTIAL LIVING, OR SHELTERED HOUSING

Congregate housing refers to arrangements in which groups of independent elderly live in separate rooms or apartments, but have various services readily available. Such housing should be constructed or renovated with the specific needs of the elderly in mind. All areas should have wheelchair access and standard safety features such as bathroom grab bars, emergency buzzers, low shelves and hand rails. The complex should also provide transportation vans, emergency medical care, some meals and resident safety monitoring.

Residents should be generally in good health, although they may use wheelchairs or walkers. They should be able to self–transfer and perform all activities for daily living independently. This type of living might be viewed as a halfway house environment between one's own home and a nursing home.

Congregate housing is not licensed by state or federal agencies, although it may be subsidized. They are often sponsored by religious groups or fraternal organizations, and units are geared to all income levels. In some instances units are condominiums, but they usually operate on a monthly rental fee like ordinary apartment rental.

The lack of a large up–front payment (except for the condominium variety, which is a recordable interest with a resale value) makes these units attractive to some individuals, but they usually do not provide medical or nursing care except on an emergency basis. If chronic problems persist to the point where activities for daily living are restricted or other health problems occur, residents are expected to make their own arrangements for additional services. Some complexes have access to the providers of homemaker and nursing services, and in some cases have arrangements with local nursing homes for possible admissions.

It is unfortunate, but to be expected, that there are long waiting lists for the more desirable and affordable of these projects. Monthly rates can range from as low as a percentage of the resident's social security check to highs of $4,000 a month or more.

An example of one of the more affluent congregate housing arrangements was a project we visited in the Northeast. This complex was located on a hundred acres of rolling land and offered alcove (studio), or one or two bedroom apartments. Each unit had kitchen facilities, private bath(s), carpeting, safety devices and maid service. Linens, van service, recreational programs and a gourmet dining room were also provided. Each day's dinner meal was included in the monthly charge, and additional meals were available at reasonable cost. A nurse was on call 24 hours a day, and they had an admission arrangement with a nearby skilled nursing facility.

The monthly fee ranged from $1,575 for the alcove apartment to $2,275 a month for the two bedroom unit. There was an additional $400 a month charge for a second individual to occupy a unit.

Senior congregate housing has recently become popular with private developers. Hyatt Hotels, for example, has formed a subsidiary called Classic Residences devoted specifically to this type of housing. Many private projects have the amenities of a fine resort hotel—with prices to match. It would seem that such residences are for the affluent.

In 1978 Congress directed the Department of Housing and Urban Development to create a low–income congregate program. Only 68 projects serving 3,000 individuals were constructed. Although the pilot program had its problems, an evaluation revealed that the residents it housed required far less nursing home institutionalization than those living in the general community. Several states have also funded congregate programs, but because of recent budget deficits, such state and national programs will not increase in the foreseeable future.

The most common complaint voiced by congregate housing residents, no matter the price of their unit, is a disappointment over the lack of kitchens by those who do not have them. Although residents in such facilities appreciate the meal service, they regret not being able to prepare an occasional meal for themselves. It is therefore recommended that this type of housing include a kitchen, provide one meal a day in the dining room and make other communal meals available if desired.

The most significant missing element in many congregate housing projects, and these include life care communities, is the lack of assisted–living (barrier–free) apartments. These small units can provide a midstep living accommodation for those elderly who have reached a point where they cannot live independently and need some protective oversight but do not require skilled nursing home care.

Congregate apartments, in tandem with the availability of assisted–living units, provide an important alternative between complete independence and a nursing home. It is unfortunate that more of these units are not available for low– and moderate–income individuals.

RETIREMENT VILLAGES
ADULT COMMUNITIES

Shuffleboard under the sun by an orange tree is the stereotypical image associated with retirement villages. This type of housing generally began in Florida, crept southwest along the sunbelt and culminated in Del Webb's Sun City, Arizona, with its 47,500 senior residents. Sun City is a giant of the genre; on average retirement villages house from 3,000 to 5,000 residents. Generally, these sunbelt communities are very activity–oriented, and direct their marketing toward younger retirees. They tend to emphasize a "resort" life–style, with lots of golf, tennis, fishing, boating and swimming. Units may be single–family homes, condominiums or mobile homes (manufactured homes not to be confused with house trailers) on rented lots.

Recent market research has redirected builders to the prospective residents' home states. They now find that most people who move from their homes prefer to stay in their own states. In the last ten years northern retirement communities have emphasized condominiums with amenities such as transportation, concierge, and security services.

Interested prospective residents should realize that each community reflects the personality of its developer and its residents. Condominium associations, community groups and building restrictions often set strict rules concerning the activities of community residents. Understand the restrictions and make sure they are compatible with your personal life–style.

The Department of Housing and Urban Development's (HUD) Section 202 Program makes direct 40-year loans to nonprofit sponsors of apartments for the elderly and handicapped. This program is tied to the Section 8 rental assistance program, whereby tenants only pay 30% of their income for housing. Under new rules their income cannot exceed 50% of the area's median income. This has barred many elderly people of modest means from these projects.

Although over 200,000 units have been constructed under this program, with only one foreclosure, it has recently been cut back out of existence. The 1991 federal budget calls for only 3,097 units. There is virtually no vacancy rate in existing 202 apartments. An average of eight people are on a waiting list for each vacancy, and this rises to 28 people for newer buildings in metropolitan areas. It is estimated that over 250,000 elderly are on project waiting lists.

State and local housing authorities have struggled valiantly with the paucity of low–cost senior housing, but budgetary problems have restricted their efforts. Only the fact that 70% of those over 65 own their own homes is cause for optimism.

Shared Housing

Shared housing is a living arrangement where two or more unrelated persons share a home to their mutual advantage. Each person has a private room and shares the common areas. There are two types of programs: matchup and group related residences. In matchup, a home owner shares with a home seeker. Group residences involve a number of people living cooperatively.

Eighty percent of the group shared residences serve only the elderly. In matchup programs, the home owner is often an elderly widow or widower with a house or apartment too large for his or her own use. The owner may desire extra income, the increased socialization due to sharing or aid in homemaking.

It is presently estimated that over half a million senior citizens are involved in such formal arrangements. Individually negotiated payment arrangements vary from fixed divisions of costs to "in kind" payments where younger individuals sharing with the elderly provide homemaker services or perform routine chores in lieu of rent. The extent and type of services performed varies, but does not include nursing care.

In order for sharing to work, a written lease must be drawn that spells out the responsibilities of each party. Many of these arrangements exist near colleges where the elderly share with students. Experience indicates that student–elder matches are more viable than elder–single parent pairings. Single parents seem to do better when they share with other single parents. In those instances they often establish mutually supportive friendships.

At present there are over 400 matchup and shared–group residence programs in more than 40 states. This is an increase from 50 such groups in 1981. Matchup organizations are usually sponsored by nonprofit groups but, unfortunately, few of the groups specifically target the elderly, even though more than one–third of the matches are with the elderly.

Various foundations have funded a national Shared Housing Resource Center that began in Philadelphia. This center was established in 1981 by Grey Panther activist Maggie Kuhn and has a complete listing of all matchup operations in the country. They are also instrumental in giving aid and instruction to newly formed organizations. The center can be reached at: Shared Housing Resource Center, 431 Pine Street, Burlington, VT, 05401. Telephone: (802) 862-2727.

There are several advantages for the elderly in shared housing: (1) it can solve financial problems, (2) it helps break the constricting ring of social isolation, and (3) it can introduce a younger person into the home who is capable of performing certain difficult physical tasks. A group shared residence has the same advantages with an even wider support group available. The difficulties in forming such arrangements are in matching the proper individuals and working out all living details before the joint residency.

Shared housing is an extremely effective means of solving maintenance, financial and socialization problems facing the elderly; it also increases the availability of residential units with little cost to society. However, it is startling to discover that the average share lasts only between 7 and 12 months, with only 8% of such relationships continuing beyond two years. It has been found that while the homeowner may desire a long–lasting relationship, the tenant is apt to be looking only for a temporary solution to a housing problem.

Shared housing is an option underutilized by senior organizations and in need of greater sophistication in its outreach and match procedures.

Accessory Apartments and Echo Housing

Accessory apartments (sometimes known as mother-daughter apartments) are self-contained living units with a separate entrance located in a larger home. They have the advantage of low cost, privacy, and yet are close to other persons who can provide support and chore services as needed.

Single family zoning regulations often prohibit these modifications, although recently many municipalities have granted variances if the apartments are occupied by elderly family members. In other localities, thousands of these dwellings exist illegally, and are usually not disturbed as long as the neighbors don't complain.

Accessory apartments are those either constructed by an elderly owner of a property or occupied by an older person. If owned by an elderly person, careful consideration should be given to the following: construction costs, which can be costly, time consuming and possibly for naught if zoning laws are violated; and, if the apartment is rented to a non-relative, landlord responsibilities, which can be a troublesome obligation for those not experienced in this area.

Initially, zoning laws prohibiting occupancy of the accessory unit by relatives of the owner seem inhuman. The overriding question, of course, is what happens to the unit when the elder occupant dies or leaves?

ECHO (Elder Cottage Housing Opportunity) housing began in Australia, where such units were known as granny flats. In Melbourne, these small portable homes were leased through the Victoria government and moved to a relative's property, where they were rented to the elderly. When they were no longer needed, they were returned to the government for reuse. Their small size kept them inexpensive, and they were accessible to a family member who could offer needed support while not infringing on the independence of the elderly person. It was envisioned that ECHO would work best in rural areas where lot size was adequate and zoning permissive.

While various groups have promoted ECHO housing in this country, and two manufactures have built these units, the concept has been limited. Lacking an effective leasing clearing house, and funding for implementation, the concept has not been viable here.

Dependent Living Arrangements

Dependent living arrangements are for individuals who need secure living accommodations with a certain amount of supervision and complete homemaker service. The resident can be mildly confused, but basically able to provide self–care.

Certain of these living arrangements can be paid for by Medicaid, if the applicant financially qualifies. Generally, this type of custodial care costs half the cost of a skilled nursing facility in any given geographic area. There are, of course, exceptions. Some rest home type facilities will take residents for a cost not exceeding a social security check, while other "posh" facilities may charge two thousand dollars a month or more.

Board and Care
Homes for the Aged, Community or Residential Care Homes, Adult Homes (N.Y. State), Retirement Homes, Rest Homes etc.

Custodial homes known as board and care facilities can range in size from those that house hundreds of residents to those that care for a handful. This type of residence is designed for the well elderly who for one reason or another are not able to live independently and who require a certain amount of supervision. The residents must be continent, not more than mildly confused, able to self–transfer and able to perform most self–care functions.

Their hotel–like service may also include recreational facilities along with other amenities. Small independent homes may offer little more than meals and lodging to their residents. All board and care facilities should provide protective oversight for their residents.

This type of facility does not provide routine health care services, and will usually require a doctor's statement that custodial care is appropriate for a prospective resident. Private and semi–private accommodations are available, and billing is on a monthly basis.

Self-pay residents may expect to pay the first month's rent plus two months security on admission. Monthly costs usually run about half of that for a skilled nursing home in the same geographic area. However, there is a wide range in cost and amenities. Luxurious board and care facilities may charge several thousand dollars a month, while others specialize in Medicaid, SSI or Social Security beneficiaries.

Many custodial facilities are sponsored by religious and fraternal organizations. Since these have an immediate socialization factor and are also aided financially by their sponsoring organizations, they tend to have the longest waiting lists.

The Problems

After the forced exodus of numerous patients from state mental hospitals in the 1970s, many of these individuals were placed in board and care facilities. There was nothing inherently wrong with such placements, if the states had provided appropriate psychiatric services in conjunction with the arrival of these new residents. Most of these facilities were not designed or equipped to be psychiatric hospitals, but many of them now house numerous residents in that category. An investigation into this type of facility should be made with this possibility in mind. Ask questions and observe accordingly.

Governmental regulation of board and care is not only spotty on a state by state basis, but also within a given state. In some instances, the only governmental control is a local health department or fire marshal.

On March 9, 1989, the late Representative Claude Pepper of Florida, who was chairman of the House subcommittee on Health and Long-Term Care stated, ". . . abuse in residential adult care centers is so broad and systemic as to be evident in every state of the Union. Neither the states nor the Federal Government . . . have evidenced any real concern for their residents' safety and welfare."

Due to weak regulation and lack of proper monitoring, residential custodial facilities in this country are in the same position nursing homes were before their regulation 20 years ago. The stories of elderly abuse that are most apt to be published today are usually connected with such institutions.

WHAT TO LOOK FOR

1. The new board & care occupant will acclimate easier if fellow residents are of similar age and interest. Check the institution's population census for age and type of infirmities. Try to avoid those centers that primarily serve psychiatric or substance dependent individuals.
2. Check with your state department of health to see what type of regulations, if any, your state utilizes for custodial institutions. Any licensing standards at all are better than no regulations.
3. Utilize the information contained in chapter five, **Evaluating a Nursing Home.** Since the rest home resident will be ambulatory and will not require nursing care, weigh the investigation to emphasize common areas, food and recreational activities.
4. A thorough credit check of the facility and its ownership might reveal potential future problems. A weak credit rating or financial problems might be a warning signal that service and food quality may be curtailed or become substandard.
5. Pay particular attention to the attitude and demeanor of the present residents. If they seem fearful or unnaturally subdued, you should immediately look elsewhere.

GROUP HOMES
PERSONAL CARE BOARDING HOMES, ENRICHED HOUSING (N.Y. STATE), DOMICILIARY CARE AND ADULT FOSTER CARE

DOMICILIARY CARE
(TERMED ENRICHED HOUSING IN N.Y. STATE)

Domiciliary care is for independent but supervised living in an apartment or house. The residents share communal meals, and certain types of other services are also provided under the direction of professional staff members who are on call 24 hours a day (it is this supervision aspect that differentiates this housing from group shared residences). This type of living arrangement can also serve the educable retarded and former mental patients, although elderly residents are usually segregated.

Payment may be made out of social security checks or on a sliding scale according to income, or the resident may be eligible for certain state and governmental entitlement programs. In areas where these programs exist, they usually operate directly under the mandate of a state agency.

ADULT FOSTER CARE

Adult foster care is a subsidized living arrangement in an approved private home. These programs are for the elderly who are capable of most self–care, but who are not able to live alone without supervision. They are often administered through a state department of social services (welfare), and operate in much the same manner as foster care for children. There are a few pilot programs that are operated under the auspices of teaching hospitals.

These living situations can provide a homey and warm atmosphere for the residents, but they are also subject to the same problems and abuses found in child foster care programs.

MONITORING

1. Due to the spotty regulation of dependent living facilities, great care must be taken by the resident's advocate to monitor the facility carefully until it is clearly established that is is adequate.
2. The resident's physical and mental condition must be periodically monitored in order to establish that the level of care is appropriate.

CHAPTER 16

MEDICARE AND MEDICAID

COVERAGE IN SKILLED NURSING HOMES, HOSPICES AND HOME CARE

GUESS WHO'S NOT GOING TO PAY?

Medicare is probably not going to pay your nursing home bill!

Prior to 1988 a Louis Harris & Associates Poll discovered that 90% of the adult population in this country thought that Medicare would pay for their nursing home costs. During the 1988 political debates concerning expanded Medicare coverage, many learned for the first time that this insurance paid a miniscule amount of total nursing home fees. The debacle over the Medicare Catastrophic Act of 1988 (since repealed) with its slightly increased nursing home benefits, lulled many people back into a complacent attitude. Certainly, they thought, what could be more catastrophic than a long nursing home stay?

Medicare only pays 2% of the total dollars spent on nursing home care (Figure 12). Medicare nursing home benefits are so restricted that only a narrow category of patient falls into their safety net, and those for only a short period of time that is usually less than the 100 day maximum benefit period.

The major limiting factors restricting coverage are: (1) the nursing home care must be provided within 30 days of an acute care hospital stay of at least three day's duration, and (2) the patient must require skilled nursing or rehabilitative services on a daily basis.

191

FIG. 12: LONG-TERM NURSING HOME CARE: WHO PAYS?

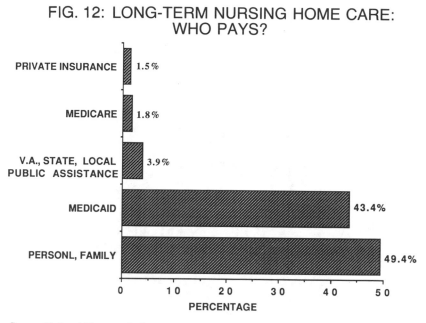

Source: National Consumer's League

A SHORT LESSON IN MEDICARE

Medicare is a federal health insurance program for people 65 or older that is run by the U.S. Department of Health and Human Services. The program is divided into two sections:

Part A: Pays for inpatient acute hospital care, some care in a skilled nursing facility, hospice care and care provided by Medicare approved home health agencies. It also includes payment for comprehensive outpatient rehabilitation facilities and outpatient physical, occupational and speech therapy.

In order to receive payment under Part A, the provider must be Medicare approved or certified. While almost all acute care hospitals are Medicare approved, only two–thirds of skilled nursing homes are, and only a third of the hospice programs.

Under Part A the facility, not the patient, submits a Medicare claim form to an **intermediary.** These are organizations selected by the government to process and pay Medicare claims under Part A. There is *usually* one designation for each state, for a national total of 60. The majority of the intermediaries are state Blue Cross groups, while the remainder are commercial insurance companies.

Part B: Pays physician's fees, outpatient hospital charges, some aspects of home care and other medical services and supplies.

Part B claims are submitted either by the patient, doctor or supplier. These claims are sent to a Medicare **carrier,** which is often the same as the local intermediary or similar group.

Doctors and suppliers can sign agreements with Medicare to become **Medicare-participating doctors or suppliers.** This means that:

1. The doctor agrees to accept the charge approved by the Medicare carrier for the service and also to take an assignment of the benefits from the patient. In these cases, there is no question that the patient saves money since the acceptable charges are always less than the usual billing for an identical service in that geographic area.
2. The doctor or supplier submits the claim directly to the carrier and is paid directly.
3. If the doctor is not a participating provider, the patient pays the full charges and submits a claim to the carrier for reimbursement according to the allowable fee schedule.

The names and addresses of Medicare participating doctors are listed by geographic area in the *Medicare Participating Physician/Supplier Directory.* You can get a list for your area by calling the nearest social security office, your state Medicare carrier or the state department of aging.

MEDICARE BENEFITS

HOSPITAL BENEFITS

After the patient pays the first $676 of a hospital bill, Medicare insurance pays the charges (semiprivate room) for the next 60 days. From the 61st to the 90th day the patient pays $169 a day. The 91st to 150 days are a one-time lifetime reserve where the patient pays $338 per day.

SKILLED NURSING HOME COVERAGE

All allowable charges in a semiprivate room for the first 20 days are paid by Medicare. From the 21st through the 100th day the patient is responsible for payments of $84.50 per day and Medicare pays the balance. There is no further coverage after 100 days.

Admission to the skilled nursing home must be within 30 days of an acute care hospital admission of at least 3 days duration. The hospital diagnosis must be related to the nursing home admission.

HOME HEALTH CARE

Payment for part–time *skilled* health care in your home for treatment of an illness if furnished by a participating home health agency and certified as necessary by your doctor is covered by Medicare.

HOSPICE CARE

Hospital insurance pays hospice care for two 90–day periods and one subsequent 30–day period. There are no deductibles except for a small coinsurance payment for outpatient drugs and inpatient respite care.

MEDICAL INSURANCE

After payment of a yearly $100 deductible, medical insurance will generally pay 80% of the **approved** charges for doctors' services, outpatient hospital care, diagnostic tests, durable medical equipment, ambulance service and certain other health services not covered by hospital insurance (Medicare Part A).

APPROVED CHARGES

Remember, **approved charges** are the fees set by the Medicare carrier, and unless your physician is a participating provider, he may charge more. Medicare will only pay 80% of the approved charge.

Durable medical equipment costing more than $150 should generally be rented.

There are a host of other major and minor exclusions to outpatient Medicare coverage. As an example, medical insurance will pay for certain diagnostic tests ordered by your doctor through an approved independent laboratory. However, many laboratories are not approved for all tests.

There have been numerous payment difficulties with the Medicare outpatient programs in the past, and some providers have reported claim rejection rates as high as 40%. The only partial solution to this problem is to deal with health care providers with good records of approval.

OTHER COVERAGE

For more detailed information on Medicare coverage, it is suggested that you call the nearest social security office for their booklet, *The Medicare Handbook*. Make sure you get a copy published in 1993 or later.

SKILLED NURSING HOME COVERAGE

In order to approve a claim for nursing home benefits, Medicare requires:

1. You have been in an acute care hospital for at least 3 days in a row, not counting the day of discharge, within 30 days of your admission to the nursing home.
2. You enter the nursing home because you require care for the condition you were treated for at the hospital.
3. A doctor certifies that you need and actually receive skilled nursing and or skilled rehabilitative services on a **daily** basis.
4. That you are not in a skilled nursing home primarily for **custodial care.**
5. That the services are actually improving your condition.

If the claim is approved. Medicare will pay for:

A semi–private room
All meals and special diets
Regular nursing service
Rehabilitation (Physical, occupational and speech therapy)
Drugs furnished by the nursing home
Ordinary medical supplies
Use of medical appliances such as wheelchairs, etc.

Medicare **will not** pay for:

Private items such as televisions and telephones in the room, hairdressing
and personal items
Private duty nurses
Extra charges for private rooms unless it is medically necessary
Custodial nursing home services provided to persons with long–term illness or disabilities

WHAT IS CUSTODIAL CARE?

Medicare legislation is very specific in that it will not pay for custodial care in a nursing home. The bulk of rejected claims concern an interpretation of what is custodial and what is skilled care. As examples, Medicare lists the following as a partial list of skilled services:

Intravenous or intramuscular injections and intravenous feedings (excepting well–regulated diabetics)

Nasogastric tube and gastrostomy feedings

Naso–pharyngeal and tracheostomy aspiration

Insertion or replacement of catheters and sterile irrigations of catheters

Application of dressings involving prescription medications and aseptic techniques

Care of extensive decubitus ulcers

Heat treatments requiring observation by skilled personnel

Initial phases of a regimen involving oxygen

Restorative nursing procedures and restorative rehabilitation (including teaching skills necessary for adherence to a regimen)

The following are considered by Medicare as supportive or unskilled functions (i.e., **custodial care**):

Administration of routine medications

General maintenance care of colostomy or ileostomy

Routine services in connection with indwelling bladder catheters

Changes of dressings of noninfected conditions

Pallative skin care, use of pallative heat, administration of oxygen after initial phases of teaching

General methods of treating incontinence

Assistance in dressing, eating and going to the toilet, assistance with activities of daily living, uncomplicated urinary tract infections (UTI) and **chronic conditions**

The interesting observation that can be made concerning Medicare's unskilled or custodial listing is that nearly all nursing homes **would never allow** even a certified nursing assistant to perform **any** but a few of the last group of nursing duties. And yet, Medicare dictates that family members and untrained personnel perform these nursing functions, even though by so doing they would be breaking the law in many states.

The federal government, while attempting to throw a sponge to the advocates of long–term care, preconditioned the coverage to make it nearly impossible for the elderly with chronic conditions to qualify. There is no question that under Medicare definitions, most care in a skilled nursing home is custodial. However, try to place that same patient in a custodial type of facility, whose cost is half that of a skilled nursing home, and find out how quickly the custodial facility will categorically reject the admission.

APPEAL, APPEAL, APPEAL

A confused patient refuses half of her physical therapy treatments and the therapist makes the proper chart notations.

Medicare withdraws benefits.

A late onset diabetic is stabilized, and the nursing staff attempts to teach him the proper way to self–administer the insulin.

Medicare withdraws benefits, even if the patient is not capable of self–administration.

Two examples of what seems like capricious determinations, but which are well within Medicare limitations. It doesn't cost anything to appeal a Medicare determination, so the byword becomes perseverance if there is the remotest chance that benefits might be awarded.

THE APPEAL PROCESS

The skilled nursing home submits the initial Medicare documentation to the intermediary (probably your state Blue Cross group). This group makes the initial determination of benefits.

If the claim is rejected, it may be resubmitted to the intermediary's reconsideration unit. This review is usually performed by a registered nurse under the supervision of a medical doctor.

If "Recon" still rejects the claim and the amount is more than $500, a hearing may be requested before an administrative law judge (ALJ). Since the ALJ has a legal rather than medical background, he often differs in his interpretations of benefit awards.

If the case is still rejected and the total amount is more than $1,000, it can be submitted to the appeals council in Arlington, VA, and then appealed to a federal court.

CENTERS FOR MEDICARE ADVOCACY

The Connecticut Center for Medicare Advocacy is a nonprofit law firm devoted exclusively to Medicare claims. They are funded by grants from the State Department of Aging and the State Department of Income Maintenance (welfare department). Their counterparts are found in other states, and their locations can be found through local aging information groups.

The states have a strong interest in establishing Medicare benefits since the more this federal program pays, the less the states will have to pay in Medicaid (a joint federal–state entitlement program) benefits.

The Connecticut group prefers to enter into a rejected case at the time of the initial turndown so that they may involve themselves in the first reconsideration by the intermediary. They claim to have a 38% success rate on reconsiderations, and an 80% success rate before the administrative judges. However, they only carry 15% of their cases before the ALJs. They have carried cases to the social security appeals council in Virginia, and won cases before the federal court (where the legal fees are paid by the government if they are successful). Most of the cases carried as far as the federal court are usually on a "class action" basis to establish a point of law.

Only 2% to 4% of Medicare participants exercise their right to appeal, although 50% of such appeals are at least partially successful.

MEDIGAP INSURANCE POLICIES
MEDICARE SUPPLEMENTS

Private health insurance companies offer Medicare supplement insurance policies (Medigap) to cover all or part of the Medicare deductibles and copayment provisions. For example, the typical Medigap policy, for an annual premium ranging from $600 to $800, would pay the hospitalization annual deductible, the $100 annual Medical deductible, and the remaining 20% of approved physician's charges.

There are several important facts to keep in mind when purchasing this type of insurance:

1. Most Medicare supplements follow the same guidelines as Medicare and do not pay if the base Medicare claim is disallowed. The 20% copayment coverage under the Medical section is only for **approved charges,** and not for the charge a doctor may make above Medicare's allowable charge.
2. These policies do not provide for long–term nursing home care. This type of coverage is granted under a separate type of policy (see chapter 18 for a discussion of long–term care insurance).
3. There have been several areas of abuse in the marketing of these policies. Some companies have sold individuals more coverage than was necessary, often with overlapping protection. There has been a certain amount of deceptive advertising in the sales of these policies.

MEDICAL–CLAIMS COMPANIES

It would seem that when any possible financial niche appears, enterprising entrepreneurs rush to fill the void. Thus it is with medical insurance claims. Private corporations have recently sprung up which offer to complete and follow up on claim procedures for the elderly. These companies charge 10% of the reimbursement when they handle Medicare and Blue Cross, and 15% for major medical claims.

These companies do not do anything that an individual cannot do, but they are familiar with claim procedures and reconsideration options, and have record keeping systems to follow the maze of paperwork. Their services might be useful for some individuals who have a large number of claims to file and who find the record keeping and procedures confusing.

Before contacting any such organization, remember that an individual need not file a claim for care obtained at a Medicare approved hospital, nursing home, hospice, home health agency, certified laboratories, comprehensive rehabilitation facilities or with participating physicians and suppliers.

MEDICAID
(KNOWN AS TITLE XIX AND ALSO MEDI-CAL IN CALIFORNIA)

Medicaid is a health care entitlement program, 56% of which is funded by the federal government, and the balance by the individual states. The program is administered by each state welfare department. Its benefits are not restricted to nursing home payments for the elderly, but our consideration of the regulations will be confined to that use.

Medicaid pays nearly half of all nursing home costs. Two out of three patients who enter a facility as self-pay, spend down their assets within a year and are forced to convert to Medicaid.

Within the general guidelines set by the federal government, individual state requirements for Medicaid benefits can vary widely. It will be necessary to contact your state about these variances.

INCOME LIMITATIONS FOR AN UNMARRIED OR WIDOWED INDIVIDUAL

The various states apply two basic financial standards to determine Medicaid eligibility. If the patient's total monthly income, from all sources, is less than the total nursing home cost, 29 states will establish Medicaid eligibility for a portion of the charges. Thirteen states have maximum monthly income limits of slightly over $1,000 a month, and 6 states have maximum monthly income levels of less than that.

While on Medicaid a nursing home patient is allowed to retain, from his monthly income, an allowance for personal needs that varies, depending on the state, from $30 to $70 a month. If that patient is deemed possibly eligible to return home at some future date, half of the states will allow a home maintenance allowance, which can range from $75 to $600 a month.

ASSET LIMITATIONS FOR A SINGLE OR WIDOWED INDIVIDUAL

Outside of the patient's primary dwelling, and a few other minor items, all but protected assets must be spent before there is Medicaid eligibility. The amount of protected assets varies from state to state, from a high of $4,000 in Rhode Island to a low of $999.99 in Missouri. Most states list protected assets at about $2,000.

Certain other assets are considered exempt, and these include household goods and personal items usually up to $2,000 in value, one wedding and/or engagement ring, a car with a value of up to $4,500, a life insurance policy with a surrender value of not more than $1,500, a burial plot and $1,500 for burial costs. Six thousand dollars in personal or real estate property can be exempt if such ownership is essential to the person's support.

Protection of the unmarried patient's primary dwelling gets rather complex within confusing state laws. Some states file a lien on the property, others will only protect it based on a doctor's certificate that the patient will eventually be discharged, while others have time limits from six months to a year.

ASSETS AND INCOME LIMITATIONS FOR MARRIED COUPLES

About the only provision that survived the demise of the recent Medicare Catastrophic Act repeal were the changes to Medicaid's spousal asset requirements. Prior to these changes, as an example, in New York State a couple with one member in a nursing home could not have more than $4,750 in assets. The new changes allow the unhospitalized spouse to retain from $12,000 to $60,000 in exempt assets. The amount exempt within this range depends on the state, but New York has used the high range of $60,000 in liquid assets, the primary residence and car. The community–based spouse can earn or have income up to $1,500 a month without affecting the hospitalized member's Medicaid assistance.

The unhospitalized spouse can keep some of her husband's income if her own is less than the set monthly fee (a minimum of $815), plus an additional amount if housing costs are greater than 30% of the monthly amount, but not more than $1,500. Special allowances are made for minor children, dependent parents or dependent siblings.

TRANSFER OF ASSETS

Benefits will be denied if a transfer occurred within 30 months of Medicaid application, or benefits will be denied for the dollar amount of the transfer divided into the average monthly nursing home rate for the state, whichever is less.

Exceptions to this rule are made for a transfer of a home for less than fair market value to a spouse, a minor child, an adult disabled child, an adult child who lived with and cared for the patient for at least two years before institutionalization, or a sibling who has an equity interest in the home and lived with the patient for at least a year before institutionalization.

MEDICAID GAMES AND WARNINGS

The transfer of assets belonging to anyone who might remotely apply for Medicaid benefits is a complex matter. Such actions should not be taken without full knowledge of the regulations of the state in which that person resides.

Care should also be taken in playing "hide the assets games." Obvious loopholes initially seem to appear in these regulations. For example, if a primary dwelling is considered an exempt asset, it might be suggested that improving that property would protect that portion invested. There are other forms of trusts and conceivable legal games, but experience in these areas is too new to say that these ploys will not be pierced by investigators.

WHO KNOWS?

Patients and their families should be aware that the nursing home staff, for the most part, is not aware of who is a Medicaid patient and who is not. They assume that private room patients are self–pay, but since Medicare only pays for semi–private rooms, and most rooms are semi–private, this distinction is meaningless. Only the most curious staff member would thumb through a chart to discover this information. The administrator's staff, the director of nursing and bookkeeping personnel are aware of billing arrangements, but it wouldn't make any difference to the others if they did know. The food is the same, nursing is identical and Medicaid also provides a monthly allowance for the resident's personal needs.

MEDICAID SCREENING

Many states now have health screening programs in addition to their financial regulations concerning Medicaid participants. The states, for cost and other reasons, attempt to keep the patients at home cared for by home health services, if it is at all possible. Beyond this type of placement screening, there are no medical restrictions concerning custodial versus skilled nursing care. Many ambulatory and continent Alzheimer's patients, as an example, are in nursing homes under Medicaid benefits.

THE CONNECTICUT ROBERT WOOD JOHNSON FOUNDATION PLAN

The Robert Wood Johnson Foundation is the largest health care philanthropy in the United States. They have recently given the state of Connecticut, and shortly several other states, a large financial grant to form a pilot program that will allow certain elderly to obtain Medicaid nursing home benefits while retaining their assets.

This program would allow the elderly to protect assets equal in value to the amount of long–term care insurance that they buy. For example, a person with total assets of $150,000 could protect $100,000 in assets by buying long–term care insurance that would cover $100,000 in nursing home costs. When that coverage was exhausted, the person would pay the next $50,000 himself and then become eligible for Medicaid even though he still had the original $100,000 in assets remaining.

This program has required special state and federal legislation and also certain commitments from the health insurance industry. It is still too early to assess the results of this pilot program.

THE TUG OF WAR
BETWEEN MEDICARE, MEDICAID AND INDIVIDUAL RIGHTS

The Robert Wood Johnson Foundation seems to recognize, as have many others, that there is something inherently unethical in requiring the provident middle–class elderly to "spend down" their assets in order to be eligible for Medicaid. With nursing home costs hovering at $3,000 a month, it does not take long for a lifetime of saving to be wiped out. The Medicaid regulations also encourage family members to play the "transfer of assets game" with their elderly members in order to avoid complete depletion of the estate.

State welfare departments want as many patients as possible on Medicare, as that relieves their budgets from onerous Medicaid costs. The nursing home industry would prefer that all patients be self–pay as those rates are higher than the Medicare or Medicaid per diem reimbursements. Patients and their families want financial relief from the burden of a long–term nursing home stay.

The federal government, caught between budgetary deficits on the one hand and the political clout of the elderly on the other, seems to grant expanded Medicare benefits while simultaneously denying their payment by strict regulations.

Everyone is in agreement that nursing home staff requirements should be increased, and that a great many other changes should be made to enhance the residents' quality of life. Everyone also agrees that there is an acute shortage of licensed nurses, and nursing assistants are a poorly paid, undereducated group performing heroically under difficult working conditions. There is no agreement as to where the funds are going to come from to correct these deficits.

This phalanx of opposing forces operates to the detriment of the nursing home resident. Nursing home occupancy is going to increase dramatically in the years to come, and it is painfully obvious that new ways to finance this care must be found.

CHAPTER 17

COSTS

DAILY RATES AND OTHER COST FACTORS

How Much A Day?

On a national average (not including Alaska and Hawaii) the cost of a semi-private room in a skilled nursing facility is $90.11 a day. It is projected that this figure will rise to nearly $100 a day by 1995. There is a wide regional variation in this cost, from a high of $117.93 in the Northeast, to a low of $78.56 in the South.

For this daily charge the patient receives room and board (usually two residents per room) and skilled nursing care on an around–the–clock basis. Also included in this basic rate are certain ancillary services such as the use of common areas and the provision of basic linens, and the expertise of such people as dietitians, recreational directors and social workers.

The per diem charge does not include drugs as prescribed by the patient's physicians, charges made for doctor's visits or the cost of rehabilitative therapies such as speech, physical and occupational. Additional charges are also levied for personal laundry, hairdressing, podiatry visits, dressings and equipment.

Some nursing homes make an additional charge for incontinent patients and for residents who must be hand fed. Additional medical services such as consultations, X-rays, dental work and eyeglass replacements will be billed separately.

It becomes readily apparent that for a patient on an uncomplicated drug regimen and with only occasional therapy, that the average daily cost will be approximately $100 a day.

Cost Variations

Nursing homes vary in cost according to the following criteria: type of ownership, type of certification, the number of beds, the region of the country, and whether or not they are in a metropolitan area.

The profit making or proprietary nursing homes are less expensive than the nonprofit (sponsored by religious or fraternal organizations) homes. Bigger is more expensive than little as the homes with less than 50 beds are less expensive than those with several hundred residents. This is probably due to the fact that the smaller homes are located in rural areas where geographic considerations keep costs lower. Skilled facilities that have Medicare/Medicaid approval are more expensive than the uncertified nursing homes since they are willing to meet the standards that certification requires.

The National Nursing Home Survey
(National Center for Health Statistics Series 13-97. These 1985 Figures Have Been Adjusted Upwards for a 5% Yearly Inflation Factor.)

Average Per Diem Rates for Private Pay Patients in Skilled Nursing Facilities

	1993	1995 (Projected)
Total	$90.11	$99.37
Ownership		
Profit making	$86.65	$95.57
Nonprofit	$98.02	$108.11
Government	$100.83	$111.20
Certification		
Skilled only	$102.96	$113.55
Medicare/Medicaid	$107.51	$118.57
Medicaid only	$86.10	$94.96
Bed Size		
Less than 50	$75.91	$83.73
50–99	$86.31	$95.19
100–199	$90.99	$100.03
200 or more	$111.51	$122.98
Census Region		
Northeast	$117.93	$130.07
Midwest	$84.27	$92.94
South	$78.56	$86.64
West	$85.99	$94.83

	1993	1995 (Projected)
Metropolitan Statistical Area (MSA)		
Met Area	$95.36	$105.18
Non–met area	$78.47	$86.54
Affiliation		
Chain	$86.71	$95.63
Independent	$92.94	$102.51
Government	$100.83	$111.20

WHY THE RATE DIFFERENCES?

PROFIT VERSUS NONPROFIT NURSING HOMES

A glance at the national average of daily rates indicates that paradoxically nonprofit homes are over 10% more expensive than profit making facilities.

The profit making institution is apt to operate under the umbrella of a nursing home chain and can reduce certain costs due to bulk purchases, insurance consolidation and other economic factors inherent in consolidated management. However, minimum state and federal staffing requirements will usually be their maximum. The Nursing Home Survey conducted by the National Center for Health Statistics found that nonprofit homes employed an average of 6.7 registered nurses (RNs) per 100 beds, compared to 4.3 RNs per 100 beds for the proprietary homes. Informal surveys on our part indicate that staffing in all departments is more extensive in the nonprofit homes.

The nursing home chain facility is responsible to its senior management who in turn must report to their stockholders. The nonprofit home will usually operate under the umbrella of a religious or fraternal organization who will have constructed a board of directors from that organization to oversee the home's operation. This board of directors is much more responsive to care complaints by members of their organization.

A good example of a nonprofit nursing home is the Masonic Home and Hospital in Wallingford, Connecticut. This 568–bed nursing home is supported by the various Masonic Lodges throughout the state, and their board of directors is made up of members from the various state districts. They provide all levels of care, including a 10–bed acute care unit. Their staffing is far and above code requirements. The facilities are such that they are used as a teaching hospital for nurses, therapists and dietitians in training. In addition to their usual charges, they receive support from the Masons and run extensive gift and endowment drives.

Nursing homes such as the nonprofit one in Wallingford provide excellent care and a sense of community. The bad news is that nonprofit homes have the longest waiting lists, and residents must usually be either members of the supporting organization or related to a member.

Although 19% of all nursing homes are listed as nonprofit, they do not all have the financial backing of the Masonic Home in Connecticut. Many are not Medicare/Medicaid approved. They tend to exist in or near the larger metropolitan areas where they can service their specific constituency.

There are still some nonprofit nursing homes that offer continuing residency on a life–care contract basis. These institutions usually offer custodial and skilled nursing care, and may or may not offer independent living quarters. They fall into a never–never land between the life care community and the typical nonprofit nursing home. The life–care contract requires the assignment of the resident's complete estate to the facility. This endowment fee (illegal in some states such as New York) is to guarantee care for life. In actual practice, the total of the patient's assets are calculated against a daily rate and when exhausted, the nursing home applies for Medicaid benefits.

GEOGRAPHIC DIFFERENCES

Nursing homes are cheaper in the south for several reasons:

> The wages are lower and there are fewer unions. In the Northeast, Local 1199 has aggressively organized many nursing homes and been successful in obtaining more realistic wages for nurse's aides and other personnel. This has not only raised wages for the union shops, but placed pressure on the unorganized homes to meet the market for labor demands. While increased union pressure combined with a labor shortage has raised costs in the Northeast, many southern states are still able to obtain some employees at or slightly above the minimum wage.
> Construction costs are cheaper in the South because of the lower cost of land, slab construction and nonunionized labor.
> Southern heating and power costs are appreciably lower.

Higher daily rates than the average for a geographic area will also be encountered in the larger urban hubs. In metropolitan New York City there is one large nonprofit nursing home that has fees totaling over $1,000 a week, and there are several corporate owned facilities that charge $1,400 a week.

The Department of Health for New York State calculates the average per diem rate for nursing homes in New York City at $160 a day, $123 a day in Westchester County and $137 a day on Long Island.

Medicare and Medicaid reimbursement rates to nursing homes set a floor on minimum daily rates (self–pay patients always pay more than this floor). Only Connecticut and Minnesota set a ceiling on maximum allowable daily rates for individual facilities. Ironically, even in these two states the most expensive nursing homes are not necessarily delivering the finest care. The individual home maximum daily rate is negotiated with the state by each nursing home on the basis of an allowable cost plus basis. This often results in a newer facility, with a high debt load of mortgage payments, charging more than an older facility with a low debt load to service. This method of establishing rates, while perhaps encouraging new construction has no correlation to either the quality of nursing care or the resident's quality of life.

AN OVERVIEW

Owners and administrators in the nursing home industry will tell you that a decent hotel room in a large city will cost $100 a day. They point out that they also provide room service without the inconvenience of tipping, full board, around–the–clock nursing care, and a complete staff of trained professionals for other services. They are quick to mention that the flat per diem rate paid by the federal government under Medicare and the states for Medicaid is a sum that is often less than their basic costs. They are dependent on the private pay patient to meet their overhead and turn a profit.

Affluent self–pay patients are able to carry this financial burden without concern. The medically indigent who qualify for Medicaid benefits are without worry. It is the provident middle class who must suffer the burden of nursing home costs which will soon average $36,000 a year. A study indicates that 46% of 75–year–olds are bankrupt after 13 weeks of nursing home care. This figure rises to 70% in one year.

WHO PAYS

Almost half of the out–of–pocket dollars spent for medical care by the elderly go to nursing homes (Figure 13). And yet, only some of the elderly spend day one in a nursing home. Obviously these costs dominate the health budgets of many older Americans.

Of the dollars collected by nursing homes, nearly half come from the resident's pockets and the other half from the Medicaid entitlement program. Medicare, private insurance and other programs make minimal payments.

OTHER CHARGES

As has been stated, there are other charges that occur in a nursing home stay. Many of these will vary according to the geographic area, and in the

FIG. 13: OUT OF POCKET HEALTH CARE EXPENDITURES FOR THE ELDERLY
By Type of Service—1984

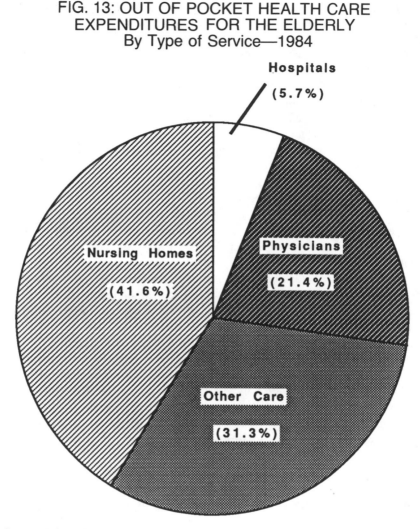

Source: National Consumer's League

case of therapies, according to the length of the session, the type of therapy and its complexity.

You may expect to pay on an hourly basis for physical, occupational and speech therapy a rate of from $35 to $55 a session. Generally, physical therapy is the most expensive.

A podiatrist, for routine care, will charge $35 to $50 for the first visit and $25 to $35 for each subsequent visit.

Hair care at the nursing home's beauty shop will be at local rates.

CUSTODIAL CARE COST
REST HOMES, HOMES FOR THE AGED,
RETIREMENT HOMES, ETC.

A careful study of the Nursing Home Survey as prepared by the Bureau of Health Statistics reveals that custodial care costs on a national average are half the cost of a skilled nursing home. An average national rate of $40 per day can be expected.

However, many of the facilities in this category are not regulated, and therefore the $40 a day figure is apt to reflect charges made by nursing homes with both levels of care rather than a free–standing rest home under private ownership. It would not be unusual for a rest home offering many social and physical amenities to charge $100 a day.

NURSING HOME CONTRACTS

At the time of admission, the nursing home administration will present to the patient or family a copy of their contract and hopefully a copy of the patient's Bill of Rights. If the new resident is a self–pay patient, they will want an admission deposit.

They are entitled to request and receive:

1. A full disclosure of the patient's financial assets. Theoretically, this will allow them to apply for Medicaid at the proper time.
2. An advance deposit. Some states have restrictions on how much of a deposit may be required. In New York State, a three–month deposit is the maximum allowed. How and when any balance in the account will be returned should be clearly defined.
3. They can require the patient or the patient's legal representative to sign a responsibility for payment form.
4. They can request to see and have a copy of an appropriate power of attorney or similar legal document.

At the time of admission the nursing home administration cannot do the following:

1. Request a donation, solicit for a building fund or use any other subterfuge to obtain additional monies for admission.
2. They cannot require the resident or his representative to waive future rights to apply for Medicare or Medicaid.
3. They cannot require a third party guarantee (responsible party) as a

condition of admission, expedited admission or a condition for a continued stay. This provision does not prevent a facility from requiring an individual who has legal access to a resident's income and assets (without incurring personal financial liability) to provide payment from such income or resources.

Note: Most of the above provisions have been mandated by the Medicare legislation, and would only apply to Medicare/Medicaid certified nursing homes. The degree to which states regulate the noncertified nursing homes varies, and in some states the facilities can demand what they wish upon admission.

How to Pay for It

At present there are only three ways to pay for long–term nursing home care: Medicaid (if you qualify), long–term care insurance policies (see chapter 18) or from deep pockets.

Life care communities, with reservations, offer an attractive alternative to this dilemma, but they are presently only available to a few. Medicare is not now, nor was it designed for, long–term care, and its strict regulations continue this philosophy. Unless the resident is medically indigent, nursing home costs will have to be paid from his assets until they are exhausted.

Home Equity Conversion
Reverse Mortgage, Sales Leaseback, Deferred Payment Loan, Reverse Annuity Loan (RAM), Home Equity Loan

Plans known as home equity conversions offer to the elderly methods by which they can tap the large equity in their homes, and yet still enjoy the benefits of occupying the dwellings.

By the time most people reach 65 or older, their largest asset is the equity in their home. Either the mortgage has been paid off, or at least paid down to a minimal amount, and the property has greatly appreciated in value. In order to tap into some of this increase in value under ordinary circumstances, the owners either have to write a new first mortgage or obtain a home equity loan (which is nothing more than a second mortgage). A new first or second mortgage, while providing capital, also requires new and higher monthly payments, which might be extremely inconvenient for retired persons on a fixed income.

Sale of the property could utilize the one–time capital gains exemption of $125,000 for those over 55, but this requires obtaining alternative housing.

Equity conversion plans have been designed for exactly this situation. Their intention is to provide a large amount of capital or monthly payments to retired individuals without requiring monthly paybacks.

These equity plans are offered by both public and private agencies. The public plans usually have income restrictions, while the private plans have no such qualifications. These plans, in all their variations, allow the owners to remain in the home and receive either monthly payments or a lump payment based on a high percentage of the property's evaluation less any mortgage or other outstanding liens. The loan is repaid when the house is sold, or from the estate when the owners die.

A variation of the RAM is the Sales Plan, in which case the owners sell the house, but retain a life estate. Some Sales Plans utilize a leaseback for a lifetime tenancy.

A split equity or life plan allows the owners to remain in the house and receive monthly payments. The purchaser owns a larger and larger percentage of the house with each payment, but does not receive clear title until some future date.

The variations and availability of these plans vary from state to state and it is suggested that you call your local area on aging or contact the National Center for Home Equity Conversion at 1210 East College Drive, Suite 300, Marshall, Minnesota, 56258.

CHAPTER 18

LONG–TERM CARE INSURANCE POLICIES

NURSING HOME INSURANCE

THE PRIVATE SECTOR'S ANSWER

The velocity of change in the last 20 years has transformed the nursing home industry. In 1970, when the average daily rate for a nursing home bed was closer to $20 a day than $100, people with modest estates did not feel that they were living under a financial sword of Damocles. As costs escalated, average stays increased and more people were assigned to nursing homes for temporary or permanent residence, financial bells rang loudly. The alarm began to sound not only to individuals, but through the corporate and governmental community. External and internal pressure was brought against the insurance industry in the expectation that free enterprise could protect us from any financial disaster.

Private insurance companies were faced with underwriting risks that tread unfamiliar and uncharted ground. They already had difficulty in ordinary health care programs, and long–term care coverage completely perplexed them because they had no firm data base upon which to build. They resisted the call.

The insurance industry felt forced to consider seriously underwriting this exposure after the late Representative Claude Pepper (Florida) of the House Select Committee on Aging insisted unsuccessfully that the federal government finance long–term care.

Back in 1984 there were 16 insurance companies issuing very restricted long–term care insurance policies. There were less than 100,000 policies outstanding. In 1989 there were 105 companies writing this type of insurance, and they had issued over a million policies, an increase of 800% (A

FIG. 14: GROWTH IN COMPANIES SELLING LONG–TERM CARE INSURANCE

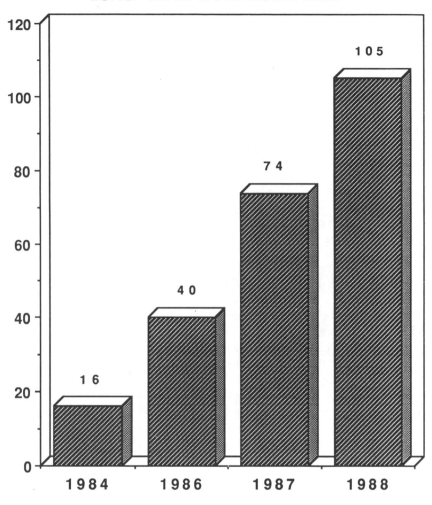

Source: HIAA, HHS, Rice & Gabel

complete list of companies issuing this insurance is included in the appendix: See Figure 14 for a depiction of this growth.

In 1989, 83% of the policies issued were to individuals, 6% to groups (almost all to one group formed by the American Associates of Retired Persons), 3% to life care communities and 8% as life insurance policy riders. Many of the largest insurers, like Aetna, only began to issue group long–term care policies two years ago.

The first generation policies in this field contained so many restrictions that they were nearly worthless. It was common for these policies to exclude coverage for Alzheimer's disease, not pay benefits for custodial or home care and not carry any provision for inflation. We are now exposed to a second generation group of policies, and the industry seems to have refined their products in order to offer broader coverage.

THE IMPORTANCE OF LONG–TERM CARE INSURANCE POLICIES

A complete understanding of long–term care insurance is necessary not only for those who might be personally interested in its purchase, but for all of those who have an interest in the problem of financing nursing home care. There are many groups and individuals who recommend private insurance as an answer to the financing of long–term care and the protection of assets for the middle class.

Several bills have been introduced in Congress that utilize this concept as part of a financing package for long–term care. The Robert Wood Johnson Foundation has awarded grants to eight states to encourage them to create a model or pilot program utilizing these policies to protect assets from Medicaid absorption. The Ford Foundation, in their 1989 report ''The Common Good—Social Welfare and the American Future,'' recommends a mix of long–term care insurance and public programs. Countless articles, editorials and interviews addressing the financial burdens of long term care have recommended private insurance as a partial or complete answer to the problem.

WHAT IS LONG-TERM CARE INSURANCE?
NURSING HOME INSURANCE

In the discussion of the insurance policies that follows, only a careful evaluation of an individual financial situation can determine if such coverage is potentially beneficial. Remember that Medicare, Medigap Insurance, Blue Cross and major medical plans do not cover long–term care in a nursing home except under very restricted circumstances.

Long–term care for the elderly can be either residence in a skilled nursing home or a custodial facility, or care provided at home. Insurance to pay for this care is written on a daily rate basis.

HOW ARE PREMIUMS CALCULATED?

Indemnity policies pay a set dollar amount per day for nursing home or home health care. The rates are fixed and do not automatically increase as the cost per day of the nursing home might. The policies are sold in increments of $10 a day benefit amounts up to a maximum of $100 to $150 a day. Premiums are also calculated according to the age of the applicant and several other significant factors:

1. Inflation riders that increase the daily rate by 5% a year usually cost an additional premium of 5% a year.
2. The deductible feature in these policies is adjusted by the number of days not covered before the benefit period begins (waiting period). This waiting period may vary from zero days to 100 days, and its length will be another determinant of the premium.
3. Some of the policies will charge a higher premium if admission to a nursing home is covered without prior acute care hospitalization.
4. Another premium variable is the number of allowable days of benefits. These policy periods can run from a year of benefits up to a lifetime.

COST

Utilizing the premium tables from a major company, we are listing below the costs for two types of coverage, one more favorable than the other:

PLAN I: $80 per day of benefits for four years with an inflation protection rider of 5% per year, and a 20–day deductible or waiting period. No requirement for acute care hospitalization.

Cost at age 50 $264 annual premium
Cost at age 60 $678.40 annual premium
Cost at age 65 $1,172.80 annual premium
Cost at age 70 $2,171.20 annual premium
Cost at age 80 $6,512.80 annual premium

PLAN II: $80 per day benefits for four years without an inflation rider, and requiring three days of acute care hospitalization within 30 days of admission to the nursing home. A 100–day deductible waiting period:

Cost at age 50 $160 annual premium
Cost at age 60 $352 annual premium
Cost at age 65 $560 annual premium
Cost at age 70 $944 annual premium
Cost at age 80 $2,680 annual premium

Home care benefits and custodial care benefits under these policies are usually half of the designated daily rate for a nursing home. Under the plans just examined, each would pay up to $40 per day for home care.

A quick glance at the premiums indicates that purchasing Plan I at the age of 80 would be financially appropriate. Sixty–five hundred dollars a year for this coverage is not sound financial planning. It might appear that purchasing the same policy at age 50, for an annual cost of $264 would be sound. If we were to predict that this 50–year–old purchaser were to go to a nursing home, we could estimate that he would do so at the age of 80, or 30 years after the purchase of the policy. Thirty years ago Medicare did not exist! Since there is no cash value in these policies, and in contemplation of possible social legislation in the next 30 years, we could not recommend the purchase of these policies that far in advance.

The age at which to consider the purchase of a long–term care policy that is actuarially viable, financially sound and politically expedient is probably in the neighborhood of 60 years of age.

WHAT THE POLICY
SHOULD INCLUDE

The long–term care insurance policy should contain the following coverage:

1. The benefits must be payable without a recent acute care hospitalization.

    Many infirmities of the elderly that can lead to a nursing home stay do not require hospitalization. Sixty–one percent of all new nursing home residents enter directly from their own home, and yet 72% of the long–term policies require prior hospitalization. These policies that provide coverage without prior hospitalization usually charge extra for that coverage.

    Home care benefits are usually at 50% of the nursing home daily rate. The policies for this care also should not require prior hospitalization. These home benefits must provide coverage for adult day care, which is a near necessity for mid–stage Alzheimer's disease patients.

2. The policy must include an inflation rider to increase the daily rate on an annual basis.

    As federal and state regulations require nursing homes to increase staffing and offer more services, the daily rates are going to increase at a velocity that exceeds normal inflation. Long–term care policies offer a 5% inflation rider, and it is probably not enough.

3. The policy must not exclude Alzheimer's disease or related disorders.

    It is estimated that 50% of all nursing home patients suffer from some form of senile dementia. Any policy exclusion for this type of affliction renders the policy worthless.

4. The length of the deductible period (waiting period) and the length of

time benefits are paid are matters for personal financial consideration. However, a waiting period in excess of 100 days reduces the value of the policy considerably. A benefit period of from two to four years will cover the majority of residents adequately.

5. The policy should clearly define the difference between skilled and custodial care.

A long–term care policy that restricts skilled care to a Medicare type definition will defeat its purpose. A custodial patient should be an individual who needs moderate supervision, but is ambulatory, continent and only mildly confused. A custodial patient is capable of almost all activities of daily living (ADLs).

PROBLEMS WITH THIS INSURANCE

The biggest problem faced in any attempt to purchase long–term care insurance is the ignorance of the average insurance agent. Agents do not seem to understand nursing homes, Medicare regulations or their own company regulations and policies. This is somewhat understandable considering most people's lack of knowledge concerning nursing homes, and the fact that long-term care policies are not only new, but evolving on a yearly basis.

The poor agents are not helped by the fact that the home offices of the insurance companies do not seem to understand their own policies. Any investigation into this topic encounters a certain amount of confusion on the part of the industry, probably due to a lack of experience factors. When asked, an officer of one major company informed us that all the data were fed into the computer, which created models upon which underwriting tables were created. We wonder where a great deal of this so called data came from? As an example, we have reliable source material which states that there are 1.5 million Alzheimer's disease patients in this country, another that says over two million, and a third, just as reliable, that says 4 million individuals suffer from this affliction. We know that nearly half of all nursing home patients have senile dementia, and yet the National Nursing Home Survey says 5.6% have senile dementia as their primary diagnosis. There are reasons for these differences, and we understand them, but it makes us wonder if the insurance industry knows something the rest of the country doesn't . . . or are they taking an underwriting flyer, as we suspect? Almost all the policies have an exclusion of coverage that reads, ''. . . expense incurred due to mental, nervous, psychotic or psychoneurotic deficiencies or disorders without demonstrable organic disease.'' In another portion of their literature they will affirm that the policy does cover Alzheimer's disease. Since no currently available test can demonstrate organic disease in a patient with Alzheimer's, one wonders at the wording of this exclusion.

We question that the industry might be straddling the fence on this issue, just in case they were swamped with Alzheimer's claims.

Many of the policies offer benefits for custodial care, but then limit their definition of this type of facility. We found it difficult to get a firm definition of custodial care facilities from the industry. The definitions provided did not fall into the parameters of most state licensuring laws and would have excluded almost all facilities except those operating in conjunction with and as part of a skilled nursing home.

Almost all policies examined were, "Guaranteed Renewable," but contained a statement that premiums can be raised if there is an across–the–board increase in the geographic area. In other words, they cannot single you out individually for a rate increase, but if they find the insurance to be unprofitable, they can raise everyone's premium in the state.

The insurance industry obviously hopes that long–term care will go the way of ordinary medical insurance and convert to group plans. Such a conversion would spread the underwriting risk across a wide age span and reduce premiums for the oldest. This seems like wishful thinking in today's economic climate. Many of our large corporations are presently faced with a massive accounting dilemma concerning present unfunded liabilities for retirees' health insurance. These same corporations are also faced with the rising cost of ordinary health insurance, and are hardly in a mood or financial position to increase employee benefits by adding still another aspect of coverage.

A 1990 report by Families USA, a Washington advocacy group for the elderly, stated that many policyholders have found their long-term care insurance useless. "There appears to be a pattern of widespread insurance industry abuse in terms of deception about what is covered and the experience people have when they file claims," said Ronald Pollack, executive director of Families USA. He went on to say that agents oversell the policies, companies deny benefits, and policyholders face delays in collecting benefits or refunds.

Several months after the report was issued, the House Committee on Energy and Commerce held public hearings on long-term care insurance. The results of those hearings verified the allegations made by Families USA.

ON THE POSITIVE SIDE

In order to better serve their policy holders, a few of the larger insurance companies are beginning to establish a network of geriatric case managers to aid in the proper utilization of nursing home benefits. If this system flourishes, it will be of great benefit to the policy holders.

Although these policies do not usually require a medical examination, there is a waiting period for pre-existing conditions.

The National Association of Insurance Commissioners (NAIC) has written a model law on long–term care policies which they have submitted to the various states for adoption. Their suggestions have now been adopted by 43 states. Adoption and policing of these guidelines by the individual states would go a long way to erasing the abuses cited by the Congressional hearing.

The NAIC recommends that states prohibit sale of policies that require prior hospitalization, and that each include an inflation provision. The model law establishes uniformity of coverage, excludes waivers denying coverage for specified health considerations, prohibits companies from offering substantially greater benefits for skilled over custodial care, and requires that all policies be guaranteed renewable.

Most critics of long–term care policies feel that the most important exclusion to coverage is that which requires a prior hospitalization. This qualification effectively bars benefits to over half of all nursing home residents.

It is important to keep in mind that new guidelines will only effect new policies, and do not cover those already in effect!

LIFE INSURANCE RIDERS

A few life insurance companies are beginning to experiment with offering long–term care coverage as a rider to their life insurance policies. Such policies will advance to the nursing home resident (or terminally ill patient) 2% a month of the face amount of the policy up to one–half of the face amount of the policy. In another instance, a policy advances 2% a month for up to 50 months.

These policies are known as accelerated–death benefit policies, and their additional cost ranges from $18 to $26 a month for a policy rider written before the age of 40, or an additional premium from 5% to 25% of the ordinary amount. As an example, a 55–year–old male taking such a policy from a major insurer might purchase a $100,000 Universal Life Policy for an annual premium of $1,836, while the accelerated–death benefit rider would cost an additional $204 per year.

At present time, there are many companies offering long–term care life insurance riders. Although the tax status for these policy benefits was ambiguous when they were first introduced, the Internal Revenue Service has now ruled that the benefits are not taxable for terminally ill patients.

In January 1990, the Prudential Insurance Company of America, the nation's largest insurer, announced that it would pay full life insurance benefits to terminally ill patients or to those permanently confined in nursing homes.

Policyholders who have been in a nursing home for at least six months and who have no expectation of discharge, can receive full benefits or elect monthly payments. No penalties would be charged except for the interest the company would have received from the money for the period. As an example, a 75 year old man confined to a nursing home purchased a $100,000 policy at age 50 and used yearly dividends to purchase paid-up insurance. This created a total death benefit of $229,340. If he turned the policy in for surrender value he would receive $163,989. Under the new program he could elect to receive $3,810 a month for 60 months or a total of $228,600.

Prudential's three million policyholders in this country and Canada will have this option as soon as the plan is approved by the state department of insurance where the policyholder resides. It is expected that other insurers will follow this competitive lead.

RECOMMENDATIONS

If you are approaching 60 and your assets are near the allowable Medicaid guidelines, those policies have nothing to offer you. Their cost on a fixed retirement income would be prohibitive, and a nursing home stay would quickly entitle you to Medicaid benefits.

If you are over 70 the cost of the coverage quickly becomes prohibitively expensive. Conversely, if you are much under 60 the coverage is cheap, but you are gambling that there will not be any significant changes in the social welfare laws in the next two decades.

Within this narrowly defined window, long–term care coverage might have benefits for your financial situation. If so, we recommend the following: (Also see the policy checklist in the appendix.)

1. Unless the insurance offered to you is written by one of the companies whose very name is a household word, check with your state Department of Insurance to see that they are qualified in your state and permitted to write this type of coverage. Go to any library and check the insurer's rating in the *A. M. Best Company Reference* volume which rates the financial stability of all insurance companies from A–plus (superior) to C (fair)). We would not accept any rating below a B.
2. An $80 a day benefit rate is close to the national average, but perhaps it should be more if you are in a high cost area. This daily rate should be protected by an inflation rider.
3. The length of the waiting period is a consideration of your own finances, but it should never be in excess of 100 days.
4. The policy must include:
   Skilled and custodial nursing home care
   Home care and adult day care
   Alzheimer's disease coverage
   Guaranteed renewability

Benefits for a minimum of two years
No prior hospitalization requirement

WHO CAN AFFORD IT?

In January 1989 the Families USA Foundation, a nonprofit advocacy group, published a study that indicated that 84% of elderly Americans cannot afford long–term care insurance policies. They also pointed out that 73% of this group could not afford even the lowest priced policy.

This study averaged premium costs for differing age groups and then struck an average from nine major insurers. They made an assumption that the policy was not affordable if its cost plus other medical expenses exceeded 10% of income.

This study differs from the 1988 Brookings Institute figures which estimated that long–term care insurance could not be afforded by 55% of the elderly.

Whichever percentage is correct, and the true answer probably lies between the two, the irrefutable fact is that a large portion of the elderly cannot afford this coverage. The answer lies in increasing the age base of the insured so that the young underwrite coverage for the old. This can only be achieved by employers including this coverage in their group medical plans. Health insurance premiums between 1986 and 1988 rose 30% without this addition, and it is doubtful that many corporations will expand coverage to include long–term care.

CHAPTER 19

THE CANADIAN ANSWER

ONE SOLUTION TO LONG–TERM CARE

A COMPARISON

The numbers are there: the elderly are increasing and more nursing home beds are needed now and in the future. It would seem as if there is going to be even less federal money to help pay for these necessities. The 1989 congressional debacle over the Medicare Catastrophic Coverage Act of 1988, which only minimally increased nursing home coverage, makes a search for other answers even more imperative. It might be revealing to take a quick look across the border and compare what Canada is doing in the area of long–term care.

Thirty–eight million Americans do not have any health insurance. All Canadians are covered by health insurance.

Universal health insurance is too costly. Canadians spend 8% of their gross national product on health care, compared to 12% and rising in the United States.

U.S. health care is better. Canadians have a lower infant mortality rate and a longer life expectancy.

A U.S. citizen can choose his own doctor or nursing home. So can a Canadian citizen.

At least senior citizens in the U.S. have Medicare. Canadian elders have no deductibles or co–payments and their programs usually pay for pre- scription drugs.

A million U.S. citizens have nursing home insurance. All Canadians have nursing home insurance.

People want to stay out of nursing homes as long as they can. Canadians have an extensive home care and homemaker system that is covered under their plan.

Canadians have to pay a daily rate for a nursing home stay, from a low of $12 a day in one province to a high of $20 in another province.

Canada has socialized medicine.

Doctors are paid for the service they deliver. Hospitals are similar to nonprofit community hospitals in the United States. The majority of Canadian nursing homes are privately owned and profit making.

Government–run programs are always expensive.

Canadian health insurance administration is 2% of the total cost. Private insurance in the U.S. costs 8¢ out of ever premium dollar to administer.

Doctors hate the bureaucracy.

Canadian doctors fill out one form that is sent to one place to collect their fees. U.S. physicians must deal with over 1,500 different health plans, and spend 10% of their office budgets on billing expenses.

CANADIAN HEALTH INSURANCE

To understand how the Canadian system works for long–term care, a brief explanation of their entire health payment system must be attempted.

The Canadians Medical Care Act of 1966 (known as Medicare), was the final refinement of their national health insurance plan. This program was formally adopted by all provinces in 1971. Their universal health insurance program is a federal–province partnership somewhat in the same manner as the U.S. federal–state partnership relationship for Medicaid. It is similar to Medicaid only in that the federal government provides more than half of the program's budget and lays down broad requirements.

Several of the major federal requirements are worth examining:

—The program must be portable from province to province.
—The program must be universal in that it includes everyone.
—The program must be publicly administered.

The remainder of the money necessary to fund the insurance coverage is raised by each individual province in methods of their choice. Some provinces use general revenue funds, others have a premium payroll deduction from employees with contributions by employers, while other provinces utilize a mix of methods. The province of Ontario, for example, has a premium payment system that costs $28.35 a month for an individual or $56.70 for a family. Each province has a system for funding the premium for the unemployed, self–employed, very young or very old.

Each province (a political division very analogous to a state) handles the program through its Ministry of Health (somewhat equivalent to a state Department of Health). The ministry establishes a yearly budget for hospitals based on past history, inflation and new programs to be created.

Doctors remain self–employed and are reimbursed by the province on a fee–for–service basis. These fees are determined yearly by negotiations between the provincial medical society and the ministry.

Acute care hospitals are voluntary (nonprofit) institutions similar to voluntary community hospitals in the United States. The patient's private doctor can act as an attending physician after the patient's admission, and be paid accordingly.

Hospital and physician's charges are completely covered under the insurance plan without co–payments or deductibles, with a few minor exceptions like extra charges for private rooms, or certain types of elective procedures such as cosmetic surgery.

Nursing homes are reimbursed by the provincial government on a patient daily rate basis. Most provinces allow a minimal daily rate charge to the patient that ranges from a low of $12 a day in one province to a high of $20 a day in another. This rate is carefully calibrated to be within the means of all pensioners and still leave each resident between $90 to $100 a month in personal funds.

Nursing homes may make an additional charge for private rooms and personal services such as hairdressers, telephones and cable television. All other fees and services including prescription drugs, therapists and physician's fees are covered by the program and the small daily rate charge.

Nursing homes are a mix of private (profit making) and nonprofit entities. In fact, United States nursing home corporations operate nursing homes in several Canadian provinces for profit. The mix of profit and nonprofit nursing homes seems to vary from province to province. In Ontario, 95% of the homes are profit making, while other provinces have a higher number of nonprofit nursing homes. The daily rate for either type of nursing home facility is identical.

The patient has a right to select a doctor of his choice, and to be placed on the waiting list of a nursing home of his choice.

A LITTLE CONFUSION OF TERMS

The Canadian federal government basically recognizes two types of nursing homes: the residential home, which corresponds to our custodial facility, and the extended care facility, which is equivalent to the U.S. skilled nursing home.

There is slightly more confusion when one looks at individual provinces, since terms differ from one to the other. Custodial homes can be known as homes for the aged, boarding homes, rest homes or hostels. Skilled nursing facilities can be extended care facilities, nursing homes, hospitals for the chronically ill or homes for special care.

As has been indicated, "Medicare" in Canada refers to the complete health insurance program rather than the U.S. program for those on social security.

The term "case manager" is also known as home care coordinator, home care case manager, placement coordinator, care coordinator, assessor or case manager. Our references will always be to case manager.

DOES CANADA HAVE SOCIALIZED MEDICINE?

Canadian health insurance is not socialized medicine any more than the United State's Medicare plan is. In a certain sense, their plan is more market oriented than Medicare since the fee for service rate between physician and the plan is at least negotiated on a yearly basis, rather than promulgated by regulation as are Medicare approved charges.

The important distinctions to remember are that each Canadian chooses his own doctor, and that the self–employed physician is paid for treatment rendered. Individuals may also choose their other health providers, including a choice of nursing home, many of which are profit–making institutions.

Although every other industrialized country in the world has some sort of national health program except the United States and the Republic of South Africa, most do operate on a socialized model. In the usual instance, the hospital facility is owned and operated by the federal, district or provincial government with a government paid house staff. Individual physicians in private practice are paid on a capitation basis, that is to say a flat sum for the number of patients on their list. As has been indicated, the Canadian Medicare program differs from these other models.

In another important respect the present system of nursing home payments in the United States is far more regulated and socialized than the Canadian model. In the U.S., 30% of all the dollars spent on health care came from the government. Half of all the money spent in the U.S. on long–term nursing home care is presently provided by the state–federal partnership, Medicaid. Medicaid daily rate reimbursements to private nursing homes is at, and often below, their overhead, forcing up the rate for self–pay patients. Medicaid also regulates payments to private physicians, pharmacists and other health providers, without the benefit of any negotiations.

Since the Canadian medical insurance plan is administered by each individual province, there are minor differences that exist. Our discussion of the plan attempts to arrive at a consensus of coverage as we perceive it.

CANADIAN CASE MANAGERS AND
LONG–TERM CARE

Medicare insurance for the elderly in the United States was designed on an acute care medical model and never contemplated treatment of chronic disease and custodial needs. As a consequence, those covered under this plan do not have true nursing home coverage, and little if any home care coverage for chronic disabilities, much less homemaker services.

Over the decades, as they gradually built and expanded their medical insurance plan, the Canadians realized that any program constructed on a strictly medical model would leave large gaps in service delivery, and in the long run would actually increase costs. Therefore, each province eventually devised a case management system for the supervision of delivery of long–term care for the elderly.

The case manager is either a registered nurse or social worker. They work exclusively with elderly individuals, except in the more remote areas where their case load may include the chronically disabled or mentally impaired. The case manager's entrance into a case may be triggered by a physician's referral, a call from a member of the family or by request of the patient.

When the case manager enters into the situation, the initial emphasis is on a functional assessment of the patient and an investigation into the availability of family care resources. At no time is there any financial means testing, although homemaker benefits for the more affluent may require a small charge. During the assessment period, geriatric assessment centers may be utilized if they are available and medically indicated. The family physician will also usually make a medical assessment either to the case manager, or in some instances directly to the Ministry of Health.

Depending on the results of the investigation into the patient's functional ability and living situation, a level of care need is assigned. This level of care may be so minimal as to require only a few hours a month of homemaker or chore services. The need may be so great as to require an immediate transfer to an acute care hospital or skilled nursing facility.

Each province, for economic and humanitarian reasons, attempts to keep the elderly in their homes rather than cause a transfer to a nursing home facility. If the assessment indicates that home care is at all feasible, the case manager arranges for the necessary services such as home nursing care, homemaker or chore service. These functions are performed by private profit making or nonprofit groups and are paid by the provincial national health program.

Case management is a continuing process. The patients (clients) are visited periodically for a further assessment that determines the increase or decrease of their level of care. Service complaints are usually directed toward the case manager for resolution.

This heavy reliance on case management has several distinct advantages:

It expands long–term care from a purely medical model which only provides for the medical requirements for those it serves to an overall view of the elderly's problems and needs.

It is intrinsic to the performance of their job that each case manager be aware of available social and medical services. This knits together the fragmentation of care so often seen in the United States.

Centralized control of programs allows for needs to be more evenly matched against resources. Needed services can be encouraged while marginal programs can be bypassed or dismantled.

Since the case manager is assigned the responsibility of monitoring individual clients, care needs can be fine–tuned and those without family or advocates do not "fall through the crack."

The case manager can act as a trained but dispassionate observer whose judgment can be respected. This is a peripheral benefit which takes away the onerous nursing home decision from the family. The case manager, knowledgeable in what appropriate care is available, can make the suggestion for nursing home residence.

It is interesting to note that in the United States, the pilot program, long–term care channeling, which is operative in certain communities in 10 states, utilizes case management and expanded services. This demonstration project will attempt to evaluate long–term costs and nursing home use under this type of system.

BENEFITS OF THE CANADIAN SYSTEM

The ability of the Canadian National Health Program to contain health care costs while providing universal coverage is an attractive feature. Aspects of their long–term coverage for the elderly also have distinct benefits which should be briefly viewed again:

Utilizing a case manager scenario, the correct services are delivered to the proper people at the appropriate time. They have recognized the obvious, that the frail elderly attempting to live independently are often the least able to search, find or afford the very programs that will allow them to remain in their homes.

As the program transcends a pure medical model it recognizes the need for homemaker and chore services. We know of several instances in our town where elders sold homes simply because they were not able to arrange or pay for such simple services as lawn care and snow removal.

Their program has removed the elderly from the devastating economic consequences of long–term care. A non–means tested health plan removes the necessity of applying for entitlement programs such as Medicaid after "spending down" all assets.

WHAT'S WRONG WITH THE CANADIAN SYSTEM?

One of the primary methods of cost containment in the Canadians system is through limitation of service. Since the implementation of the 1971 revised laws, acute care hospital beds have decreased. In some areas, long waits for elective surgery have been reported. In another province, admission to a skilled nursing home may take as long as a year.

In most provinces, nursing homes operate at 97% of capacity, which means that at any given time there are no available beds. New construction of nursing homes is carefully controlled and limited by each province.

Although one province requires a five day turn–around for its assessment program, other areas have waits for as long as six months before a long–term care assessment is performed.

A strong case management system has many benefits, but it has a dangerous loophole when the case manager is also the "gatekeeper" for services. If cost containment becomes necessary, subtle pressure can force a downward movement in assessments and the subsequent delivery of services.

Although Canadians are as interested in nursing home quality of life as the rest of us, their inspection and monitoring systems are far more loosely organized than in the United States. Massive governmental regulations, such as exist in the U.S., simply are not promulgated in Canada. Unannounced nursing home inspections are made, but they are "not unexpected." They seem to attempt to solve deficiency problems by suggestion rather than confrontation. This friendly attitude may work in a country with a small and homogeneous population, but would require extensive revision if transported into the U.S. with its history of entrepreneurial zeal.

PHYSICIANS FOR A NATIONAL HEALTH PROGRAM

In the United States, a group called Physicians for a National Health Program is headquartered in Cambridge, Massachusetts. It has several thousand members and promulgates a system very close to the Canadians model.

An examination of their proposal, as published in the January 12, 1989, issue of the *New England Medical Journal,* indicates that they favor adopting nearly all of the Canadian program.

This group suggests that a national health insurance program be initially tested in several statewide demonstration projects. Similar to the Canadian federal–province partnership, they envision a federal–state meld. The plan would be publicly administered, universal and cover all medical services including long–term care and home care. All other insurance plans, co–payments and deductibles would be abolished.

The plan suggests a fee–for–service payment system to doctors, although it also anticipates physicians in salaried positions within group practices or health maintenance organizations (HMOs). Hospitals would be financed on a yearly budget basis.

The plan would pay the present owners of profit making hospitals, nursing homes and clinics a fair return on equity. Future capital investments would be made by the program.

Their specific program for long–term care has not been delineated at this point, but it is anticipated that they will endorse home care, a strong case management system and nursing home coverage.

COULD NATIONAL HEALTH INSURANCE BE ADOPTED IN THE U.S.?

The public versus private battle over health care costs has now been going on for over 40 years. It was President Franklin Roosevelt's intention to introduce a health care bill into Congress, and in 1945 Harry Truman called on the Congress for such legislation. In the early 1970s the Nixon administration prepared a hybrid bill for national health insurance, and in his first address to Congress in August of 1974, President Ford asked for passage of national health insurance.

Recent conservative attitudes, combined with the large national budget deficits, would act against any program with costly start–up costs.

The special interest groups to fight against this type of legislation would be formidable. Any viable type of national health insurance plan precludes private sector insurance. The insurance companies, with their untold billions in assets, would oppose any such enabling legislation. The large for–profit corporations now involved in hospital, nursing home and clinic ownership, would also fight such action. It could be reasonably expected that the conservative nature of the American Medical Association would earmark that group as a powerful member of the opposition.

The remainder of corporate America, after a good second look, could probably be induced to support national health insurance for their own economic gain. Although employers would still be expected to make reasonable contributions to the program, it would result in large financial savings for individual corporations. It would also relieve these companies from their present acute adversarial relationships with employees and retirees concerning payment for and expansion of health benefits.

The 38 million Americans who presently do not have any health insurance are mostly the poor and the very young. They speak in quiet and unsophisticated voices. Their elders, as the congressional reversal of the 1988 Medicare Catastrophic Act surcharge proved, speak with an effective voice. This constituency, already partially protected by Medicare, and only needing a few elements incorporated into the program, such as nursing home and prescription drug coverage, would be a resounding voice for its adoption.

The AARP, in a 1990 informal survey of 70,000 of its members, found that 84% called for a government-sponsored national health insurance program.

CHAPTER 20

CONCLUSION

A SUMMARY

The typical nursing home resident is an 82–year–old widow who is not able to bathe or dress without help. She has difficulty either seeing or hearing, and experiences one or more chronic medical problems. She will live for two and one-half years in a building where half of the other residents are incontinent, and another half have some form of senile dementia.

These people are obvious candidates for constant care, and are not warehoused for the convenience of venal or lazy relatives!

In 1939 there were 1,200 nursing homes in the United States, 9,000 in 1950 and 27,000 in 1989. This explosive increase in the number of facilities would seem to reflect the rise in our aged population (Figure 15), but a 90% occupancy rate indicates that this dynamic addition of beds is still grossly inadequate.

For financial and humane reasons, home care has been encouraged. It is unfortunate that this emphasis has operated in a near vacuum of proper support services in the form of case management and delivery. Existing home services are in disarray with a paucity of competent individuals to deliver such care. Although some geographic areas have a network of care services for the elderly living at home, they are often fragmented and confusing to obtain without professional guidance. In other areas, certain services may exist, while others are impossible to obtain within the financial reach of most frail elderly.

Some elderly are erroneously domiciled in nursing homes due to their advocate's ignorance of available alternatives. Others of the frail elderly are loyally kept home to their physical and psychological detriment. Often these cases cause devastating problems to the family structure of those attempting care under heroic circumstances.

Nursing homes are not going to go away! Although they do it poorly, they serve an important medical and social need in our society. It is incumbent on the patient's advocate to select the best of the available homes, and to monitor care closely during the resident's stay. It would also be helpful

FIG. 15: THE GROWING ELDERLY POPULATION I MILLIONS (2000 IS AN ESTIMATE)

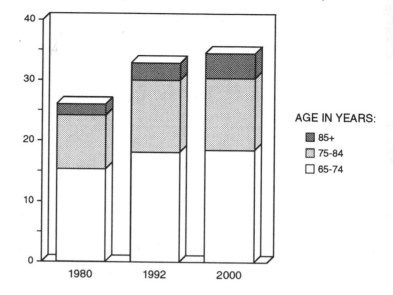

AGE IN YEARS:

■ 85+
▨ 75-84
□ 65-74

1980   1992   2000

Source: Census Bureau

if these same individuals actively worked toward improving long-term care for the elderly in any manner they could.

As we all age, the probability of our own nursing home residency increases proportionately. We address our own future when we actively pursue improvements in nursing homes.

PROBLEMS OF THE NURSING HOME INDUSTRY

A discussion with any nursing home administrator, at anytime, in any locality, will develop a similar list of industry problems. They all voice the same complaints: They are convinced that they operate in an over–regulated industry pressured by impossible societal and medical demands; they are forced to work within the confines of constantly decreasing profits complicated by extreme personnel problems.

While it is true that state inspections often have a "Mickey Mouse" quality, those standards are the only means to provide a modicum of consumer protection to the resident. Inspections do turn up serious deficiencies that are occasionally serious enough to cause the loss of licensure. The industry fails to acknowledge that over two decades ago they were in such disarray, without self–policing mechanisms, that they brought state and federal codes down upon themselves.

A cursory observation of nursing home patient advocacy groups and possible new legislation and regulations reveals that there are strong demands for increased nursing home staffing. Missing from these demands are the provisions to pay for these increases. In many areas, Medicaid payment for patient care is at or below the operating cost of the facility. And yet, these payments account for half of the monies the industry receives. Any increase in staffing must be funded by self–pay patients or Medicaid. Neither alternative is acceptable to those who pay nursing home bills, or to those who pay the taxes which support Medicaid.

If funds are somehow provided for increased staffing, where are they going to find the people to fill those slots? At the present time, one in three nursing homes report severe shortages of registered nurses, and 40% report a moderate shortage. Twenty–three percent of all nursing homes have a severe shortage of licensed practical nurses, while 56% have a moderate shortage. Nurse's aides are in equally short supply, and these shortages are under present staffing requirements!

It is estimated that the country presently faces a shortage of 500,000 registered nurses. Nursing school enrollments have dropped so severely that many nursing schools have either closed or drastically reduced class size. In addition, geriatric nursing is far down the preference scale for recent nursing school graduates. There are also shortages in other health care specialities such as dietitians and all types of therapists.

Patients and their advocates often complain of verbal abuse by nurse's aides. In low unemployment areas, nursing homes are forced to hire and attempt to train literally anyone who walks through the door, merely to adhere to code requirements.

Nursing homes, as are all health care facilities, are labor intensive. A rough rule of thumb for personnel is one employee for each patient bed. This includes not only nursing personnel, but maintenance, food service and clerical help.

Nursing home personnel shortages are further exacerbated by two additional pressures: To curtail costs and adhere to diagnosis related groups, acute care hospitals are discharging sicker patients to nursing homes; and some states are establishing Medicaid nursing home waiting lists by level of care. In both instances, frailer patients enter nursing homes without any increase in staff requirements.

Sophistication of management and centralization of purchases and other cost containment factors are seemingly not the answers to nursing home fiscal problems. Beverly Enterprises, Inc. of California is an example. Starting with 47 nursing homes in 1971, by 1986 Beverly owned 1,136 nursing homes in 45 states and Canada. They were the leader of the industry until the bubble burst. A staff turnover of 78% a year, Medicaid rates as low as $37 a day and overexpansion forced them into deep problems by 1988. In 1989 they sold off large groups of their property and withdrew completely from several states. In 1988, the nation's seventh largest nursing home chain, Care Enterprises of Tustin, California, filed for bankruptcy.

What's Wrong with Those Damn Nurses?

In our discussion of choosing and evaluating a nursing home, we stressed the importance of adequate staff, its competency and attitude. We categorically stated that personnel are the keystone to good care. It is the weakness of this keystone that casts a dark shadow across the nursing home industry and more importantly, the residents.

Geriatric nursing is not only one of the most physically taxing positions in the nursing field, it is the worst paid, the least emotionally rewarding and the job most likely to expose the staff to physical and verbal abuse. The nature of the work makes it the least pleasant of nursing functions.

Good nursing care requires a constant repositioning of patients, transfers, from chair to bed to toilet, bathing and help with other functions. Some transfer patients are not only immobile, but can be large and uncooperative. When moving patients in an acute care hospital, a nurse can call on an orderly or another nurse. For the most part, nursing homes do not have orderlies, and other nurses are often not available. Without exception, nurses in this field suffer back problems. It is not unusual to see a slight, 100–pound female nurse or aide transfer a 200–pound male not once but several times during a shift. Male aids and nurses in the nursing home are a needed but rare and precious commodity. Rank does not have privilege. If aides are not available, licensed practical nurses and registered nurses must do what must be done.

Any licensed nurse can earn far more in an acute care hospital or working private duty through a registry. Nursing assistants, unless they are unionized (a rarity), are paid from $.50 to a $1.00 an hour more than wages given teenagers at the local fast–food establishment. There is no career advancement available for aides and licensed practical nurses. Career potential for a registered nurse in a nursing home is quite limited. Caught within the confines of their job descriptions, nursing personnel are rewarded with minor cost of living salary increases or minute increments granted for longevity. The youngest RN on the floor is making nearly as much as the most experienced.

There is a lack of emotional rewards. It is true that many members of the nursing home staff become truly fond of their patients, but the joy of participating in cure and recovery is not present when dealing with the chronically ill elderly. Eventually, most nursing home patients will decline in function.

Contrary to popular belief, that sweet, frail, great–grandma can pack quite a wallop. Confused patient's are often both physically and verbally combative. The nursing home staff is more vulnerable than a psychiatric nurse to unprovoked attacks because the physical transfers that must take place expose the nurse or aide to assault. It is not a question of *if* a nurse will be hit, it is a question of when and how often. Luckily, the fraility of the average patient reduces the potential for harm. Verbal abuse is expected from some patients, and inappropriate sexuality is also occasionally present. Trained geriatric personnel learn to cope, but the ill–trained often react, and another case of patient abuse is documented.

Nurses expect to experience the good and the bad in their profession. In geriatric nursing, the scales seem tilted toward the negative. In any skilled nursing facility, half the population is incontinent, half are confused and many are comatose, aphasic, terminal or with other conditions not faced by a staff dealing with exuberant new mothers in a maternity ward.

New opportunities for women have been devastating to the nursing profession. The brightest potential nurses have either gone on to medical school or opted for newer opportunities in a host of other professions that provide greater independence and career advancement. Condescending attitudes by some male physicians toward nurses has not encouraged the profession.

In addition to the litany of complaints listed above, the nursing staff must daily face a population that does not want to be where they are. They are also confronted by family visitors ridden with guilt, who are convinced that the nurses are abusing their relative. They work in understaffed facilities, which means that they are not able to perform their duties properly. They often know they are only providing minimal care.

But it is the nurse's aides who spend the majority of staff time with an individual patient. We are entrusting the most fragile members of our society to poorly trained individuals who are paid only slightly better than young teenagers serving hamburgers. We demand legislation to guarantee a more significant quality of life for our nursing home residents, without provision for either the emotional support or economic benefits to the unskilled members of our society who are ultimately responsible for this care.

How to Make the Field More Attractive

The Nurses

Attracting bright and compassionate male and female students into the nursing field, and their subsequent dedication to geriatric medicine, is a problem of huge dimensions. We are not faced with a national shortage of physicians, but do have an extreme shortage of nurses. Tuition remission programs, increases in starting salaries and improved working conditions are a beginning, but not the complete answer to this problem.

Every complex society has always had a number of critical professions which were essential. Circumstances often dictate that these professions are not the highest paid, and so a certain mystique grows around their desirability. The income of a lawyer in private practice is far higher than a judge. Military and police officers have never enjoyed high salaries, but those callings still attract dedicated individuals. Many of our brightest students enter teaching out of love rather than financial return. We must create this mystique around geriatric nursing so that it becomes a profession aspired to, rather than a job settled for.

Anyone who has ever lived with a high school senior during their last months before college is aware of the massive recruiting efforts mounted by the military. Brochures deluge the mailbox, while well groomed sergeants call and cajole until it seems as if joining the navy or army is a necessity for any right thinking young person. If we can mount this type of campaign for the military, can we not do half as much for a profession that will affect all of us when we are the most in need?

Nursing Assistants

At the present time, a nurse's aide or nursing assistant is an unskilled employee whose training has consisted of a few hours of classroom time and a few days of clinical "on the job training" at her place of employment. There is no potential for advancement whatsoever! As a consequence, the field is populated by high school dropouts, marginal employees and for the lucky nursing home, individuals who would rather do that work than the repetitive tasks of a factory assembly line.

We propose a network of teaching nursing homes that would train ambitious aides for a limited nursing license. These teaching facilities would utilize existing units, and they would grant certificates to licensed geriatric practical nurses. Individuals in these programs could be either high school graduates or holders of GED certificates. They would work and be paid for full–time aide duties while also attending class and receiving clinical instruction. This work–study relationship would require longer programs than an ordinary licensed practical nurse course, but the specialized nature of the instruction would allow completion within a two year period. This viable career alternative would direct a stream of trained individuals into the field, and allow single parents and high school dropouts to earn and learn simultaneously. Geriatric practical nurses, because of their license limitations, would continue working at nursing homes, or be available for similar duties with home care agencies.

A similar but more complex program could be instituted to allow experienced licensed practical nurses to upgrade their licenses to geriatric registered nurses.

The use of these two innovative programs would construct a career ladder that led from untrained nurse's aide to geriatric practical nurse and subsequently to geriatric registered nurse.

A NEW JOB DESCRIPTION

We further propose a new employment category to be called geriatric health aide. These individuals would be drawn from the ranks of the active elderly. They would be part–time employees who would receive wages equivalent to the amount they could earn without disturbing their social security benefits.

The health aide would receive 40 hours of orientation and training, and would be utilized for certain care functions and companionship with nursing home residents. They would assist in patient grooming, feeding and other non–nursing or non–aide functions. In essence, their position would be more social than medical as they would spend their daily hours with two or three residents. This new category of employee would not only relieve the nursing staff of some functions, but would enhance the quality of life for many lonely residents.

PROBLEMS WITH THE DOCTORS

Only 150 physicians a year complete fellowships in geriatric medicine or geriatric psychiatry. There are not more than 700 doctors in the country who have completed training in these sub–specialties, and yet the over–65 population takes up 36% of all physician's time and accounts for 40% of acute care hospital days. Most physicians learn geriatrics by default since so much of their practice is composed of the elderly. Formal geriatric training, however, inculcates a sensitivity to the unique problems of the elderly, and experience alone is an inadequate substitute.

Care of the elderly is not glamorous. It does not provide for the possibility of a miraculous cure. It is time consuming. A physician with a heavy Medicaid practice is not wealthy. One state pays doctors as little as $9 a visit for their Medicaid patients. Economic and poor medical prognosis has dampened the interest of physicians in the practice of geriatric medicine.

This situation is dramatically revealed in the paucity of research into many areas of elderly medical problems and care. At the beginning of chapter 11 we stated that on any given day several hundred thousand of our elderly are physically and chemically restrained. We further postulated that restraints were the single most significant factor in nursing home patient abuse. The sheer numbers involved and this potential for abuse would seem to signify the dramatic importance of this topic. And yet, the research and publication of scholarly articles on this subject is practically nonexistent. A 1989 article in the *Journal of the American Geriatric Society* which surveyed the literature on physical restraints found "With elderly nonpsychiatric patients only ten studies of physical restraints were found."

Ten! In most other areas of medicine a topic of this significance would have produced hundreds of published research studies. This is only one example of the lack of research into the problems and care of the fragile elderly.

SOLVING THE PROBLEMS WITH THE DOCTORS

An increase in the number of physicians trained in geriatric medicine is an essential problem that is easily solved: we buy them!

A yearly budget to attend a private medical school is about $27,000, and perhaps a third less at a state supported university. Medical students have three options to finance this: they pay the cost from family funds, they make an extensive commitment to the military or they borrow. Loan money is available for training doctors, and it is not unusual for a new physician to graduate with a debt load of over $80,000. This method of financing new physicians discourages entrance into the lower paying specialties such as academic medicine, pediatrics, psychiatry or geriatric medicine.

Providing a loan remission program for new physicians who specialize in primary care, which would include geriatrics and academic medicine, would attract a host of bright new doctors with an idealistic calling. If we concurrently provide more grant money for research in geriatrics, these newly trained geriatricians would apply for and perform the basic studies we so desperately need to care for nursing home patients.

WHAT ELSE MUST BE DONE?

If it is at all practical, for economic and emotional reasons home care is preferable to a nursing home. We fear that available resources, specifically trained people, are not adequate in number and experience. The nature of this shortage is heightened by the lack of a case management system to direct resources and identify need. Until adequate numbers are recruited into the various layers of nursing tiers, there are just not enough people to staff nursing homes and provide home care service. As long as existing personnel must be economically marshaled, it must be considered that a nurse on the unit floor is more effective than the one in an automobile traveling from house to house to deliver one on one care.

We fear that many people truly in need of a skilled nursing home do not obtain it because of a universal distaste for the concept. The time may arrive when we can provide adequate health care personnel for both the home and the medical facility, but until that time arrives, let us make the nursing home milieu as attractive as possible. In order to help do so, we recommend the following actions to be instituted as soon as possible:

GOVERNMENT REGULATIONS AND INSPECTIONS

At the present time, state inspection teams that monitor nursing homes are primarily concerned with the physical welfare of the residents. Admirable as this is, it is not a holistic approach that takes into consideration morbidity factors due to the lack of psychological well–being of the residents. These inspection teams must be expanded to include selected "visiting members" from the industry and lay public.

It is recommended that members of family councils from other nursing homes, administrators of out–of–state nursing homes and selected members of the retired community be placed on these inspection teams. These individuals, knowing the tricks of the trade, or able to engage in intimate dialogue with the residents, might obtain information more useful than the number of swabs in a medicine chest.

The time lag between the discovery of gross deficiencies and the loss of license or state takeover should be shortened. Stiffer financial penalties for other deficiencies should be levied.

Government regulations should increase staff coverage per patient hour, and encourage rewards for over compliance in order that the minimum does not become the maximum as is so often now.

As several recent fires prove, patient safety can be increased by requiring sprinkler systems in all nursing homes. No waivers should be granted for age of construction or other factors. Although winter temperatures are closely monitored, no requirements exist for air conditioning. We have seen too many patients with pulmonary problems expire prematurely in the summer due to excessive heat and humidity. If we can air condition our retail shops, we can our nursing homes.

Regulations should be immediately implemented to insure that all custodial and rest home type facilities fall under stringent licensing and inspection requirements. Inspections of these facilities should be as tight as those performed on the Medicare/Medicaid skilled nursing home.

NEW FACILITIES

At the present time nursing homes operate at 90% of occupancy. This means that some patients remain in home high–risk situations, or stay in acute care hospitals longer than necessary. Institutions that are filled to near capacity cannot offer families temporary respite care, "sample stays" for those considering nursing home admission or wards for short–term hospice type units. High occupancy rates reduce the consumers' element of choice and do not allow normal market competition to increase care. Today's lack of adequate facilities does not even begin to contemplate the future expansion in patient numbers as the number of elderly increase.

Although we obliquely criticize Canada for containing costs through limitation of services, half of our states have "certificate of need" qualifications for capital expenditures for hospitals and nursing homes. Governmental authority well realizes that for every two nursing home beds created, at least one will be occupied by a Medicaid patient. "Certificates of need" restrictions must be viewed in a light other than cost containment.

Innovative developers and operators of nursing homes should be encouraged. Low cost construction loans and low interest permanent loans would do this. Individual communities could utilize selective zoning and tax abatements to entice this construction to the proximity of retirement villages, low cost housing for seniors or congregate housing.

Nursing homes should be constructed near where senior citizens presently live. This would allow for viable day care programs, health maintenance and a continuity of care.

Dedicated Alzheimer's units staffed by highly trained personnel should be an integral part of each facility. Geriatric assessment centers must be integrated into acute care hospitals in such numbers as to be reasonably accessible to all members of our population.

Nursing homes are presently designed to resemble acute care hospital models. Sterile halls with nursing stations located at appropriate locations reek more of hospitals than any pretense of residential living. The sterility of these buildings indicates a complete lack of architectural or artistic flair. They seem built to adhere to minimal regulations and low construction costs rather than any resident's aesthetic needs. It would be interesting to see what innovative designs some of the architectural talent available in this country could devise for nursing homes if they were to receive such assignments.

IN CONCLUSION

We envision a health care and social services delivery system for the elderly that is available to everyone. This program would provide knowledgeable medical care backed up by a full range of pharmaceutical, ocular and dental services.

Supervised by trained case managers, nursing, homemaker and chore personnel would strive to keep older persons in their homes for as long as possible. This same network with the addition of adult day care centers, adequate respite care and more professional help would aid families who attempted to care for their frail elderly.

If long–term nursing home care were necessary, it would be provided at affordable cost. Residents would have a choice of light, airy, home–like facilities. These institutions would be staffed in adequate numbers by people dedicated to the profession of geriatric care.

Nursing home residency would not only attempt rehabilitation and stabilization of the patient, but would concern itself equally with a fruitful existence within life's continuum.

GLOSSARY

Actual Charge (Medicare related) is the amount a physician or supplier actually bills a patient. The rate paid by Medicare insurance may differ.

Acute Care Hospital is the general term for community hospital, general hospital or teaching hospital.

ADLs are the activities of daily living, such as grooming, eating, dressing, etc.

Aging is the process by which structural changes accumulate with the passage of time, not due to disease or accident.

Agnosia is the inability to recognize people or things.

ALJ refers to administrative law judge, who may hear an appeal for a rejected Medicare claim that is more than $500 and has already been reviewed by a Reconsideration Unit.

Alzheimer's Disease is a progressive, terminal form of dementia that is diagnosed by exclusion. Its cause is unknown. (See **SDAT**)

Ambulation means to walk, either independently or with assistive devices or support.

Ambulatory is the ability to move around at will.

Ancillary Services (in a nursing home) are those services other than room, board and professional medical services.

Aphasia is the inability to communicate because of a brain defect in speech, comprehension, reading or writing.

Approved Charges is the amount of money Medicare approves for a particular service rendered, rather than the amount charged by the physician.

Apraxia is the loss of purposeful movement.

Assignment (Medicare related) is the process by which a doctor or supplier agrees to accept payment directly from Medicare.

Atherosclerosis refers to the narrowing and hardening of arteries. The cause remains unknown. (See **Coronary Artery Disease**)

Atrophic Urethritis (in women) is a wasting of tissue comprising the urethra, a canal leading from the bladder used for the purpose of discharging urine. This condition predisposes an individual to urinary incontinence.

Attending Physician is the physician who is medically responsible for the patient.

Autoimmune Diseases are disorders whereby the immune system attacks the body's own tissues.

Cardiac Care Unit (CCU) is an intensive care unit for patients whose primary problem is heart disease.

Carrier (Medicare related) refers to a private insurance company under contract to the federal government to process physicians' and suppliers' Medicare claims.

CAT Scan refers to computerized axial tomography which is essentially an x-ray that permits detailed examination of a tissue, such as the brain.

Catheter refers to any hollow tube that permits administration (or removal) of substances to a patient. (See **Foley Catheter**)

Cerebrovascular Accident (CVA) is the medical term for stroke.

Charge Nurse is the nurse assigned for a given shift to be the nurse "in charge." Charge Nurses should be aware of the status of each patient on their unit.

Chart is the patient's medical record.

Chronic Disease is a disorder which persists for a long time and is commonly permanent or disabling.

Chronic Obstructive Pulmonary Disease (COPD) is a general term for diseases of the lung such as chronic bronchitis and emphysema.

Clinical Depression is a term some physicians will use to describe patients whose moods are depressed; it is not a medical diagnosis. (See **Depression**)

Code consists of a specialized medical team's response to a patient who has stopped breathing or whose heart has stopped. The response includes, but is not limited to, CPR, establishing an artificial airway with a breathing tube, administration of medications and artificial respiration.

Cognitive Function is that aspect of brain function concerned with thought, reasoning and perception.

Colostomy is a surgically made opening in the abdominal wall through which stool passes. A colostomy is covered by a plastic bag (colostomy bag) which is changed or emptied when filled with stool.

Comatose is the state in which a patient is unconscious and cannot be aroused. Patients who are comatose also lack the ability to open their eyes spontaneously.

Confusion is a symptom common to several disorders and is characterized by impaired memory and alertness, disorientation and diminished intellectual capacity.

Congestive Heart Failure (CHF) is a condition in which the heart is unable to pump blood adequately into the blood vessels because of a weakening heart muscle. It is characterized by shortness of breath and ankle edema.

Congregate Housing is elderly housing which provides at least one meal a day in a common dining room and other assistive services.

Conservator is a court–appointed individual empowered to act on behalf of another.

Contracture is an abnormal shortening of the soft tissues of a limb which causes it to be permanently fixed in a rigid position.

Coronary Artery Disease (CAD) refers to atherosclerosis of the blood vessels of the heart. (See **Atherosclerosis**).

Custodial Care includes room, board and protective oversight delivered on a long–term basis without routine medical or nursing services.

Decubiti (pressures sores, bedsores) are ulcerative lesions that occur over pressure points.

Dedicated Dementia Care Unit (DDCU, Alzheimer's Units, Confused Patient Units) is a separate facility in a skilled nursing home for patients with dementia.

Delirium is a reversible form of confusion characterized by an altered state of alertness, forgetfulness, hallucinations and incoherence. Common causes of delirium include infections and medications.

Delusions are false beliefs inconsistent with reality, such as believing that you are Julius Caesar, a delusion of grandeur.

Dementia is an irreversible disease process that causes confusion and deterioration in cognitive functioning.

Depression (Major Depression) is a diagnosis rendered by a physician and is characterized by, but not limited to, loss of interest in life, apathy, weight loss, sleep disturbances and feelings of worthlessness. (See **Clinical Depression**)

Diabetes is a condition in which the body is unable to metabolize sugars (carbohydrates) properly. Patients with diabetes can experience hyperglycemia if their condition is untreated or poorly controlled.

Diagnosis by Exclusion refers to disorders which can be diagnosed only after excluding other conditions.

Diagnosis Related Group (DRG) is a grouping of various medical conditions for the purpose of determining the hospital reimbursement rate.

Dialysis (esp. Hemodialysis) is a therapy used for patients with chronic renal failure. Blood is pumped from a patient through the dialysis machine, where waste products are removed, and back to the patient.

Discharge Planner an individual, usually a social worker or registered nurse, in an acute care hospital or nursing home who aids in the planning and placement of discharged patients.

Diuretic is a medication—such as Lasix or thiazides—that promotes the production of urine. Diuretics are commonly used in the treatment of hypertension and congestive heart failure.

Domiciliary Care refers to a type of shared living arrangement that is communal in nature. A professional manager or superintendent is usually present.

Do Not Resuscitate (DNR) is a type of order written by a physician which limits heroic measures to be performed on a patient in the event of a cardiac or respiratory arrest.

Edema is the excessive accumulation of fluid in the tissues, commonly manifesting itself as swollen ankles.

ECHO Housing (Elder Cottage Housing Opportunities) small homes in which elderly individuals reside, which are constructed on the property of another individual.

Emphysema (See **Pulmonary Emphysema)**

Ensure is a common liquid formula nutritional supplement and is usually given through feeding tubes.

Falls occur when a person unexpectedly drops without any known cause.

Feeding Tube is a hollow tube through which liquid nutrients and medications may be given.

Foley Catheter is a hollow tube passed through the urethra into the urinary bladder to facilitate the passage of urine.

Frail Elderly is that group of the geriatric population at highest risk for injury or debilitating disease.

Functional Status is the degree to which a person can perform ADLs.

G-tube (Gastronomy Tube) is a feeding tube that has been surgically placed through the abdominal wall and into the stomach.

Gastroenterologist is a physician who has specialized in the disorders of the GI tract, which includes the liver, pancreas, stomach and intestines.

Geriatric Assessment Unit is a hospital clinic, usually in a large medical center, staffed by individuals knowledgeable in geriatrics who are capable of providing complete functional, physical, neurologic and psychologic evaluations of a geriatric patient.

Geriatric Chair (Geri–chair) is a padded chair with small wheels and a high back designed for support.

Geriatrics refers to the health care field that deals with the problems and diseases of the elderly.

Gerontologist is a physician who has specialized in gerontology, the scientific study of the problems of aging in all its aspects.

Gingival Hyperplasia is the medical term for swelling of the gums.

Group Home is a shared living arrangement.

Guaranteed Renewable is an insurance company agreement to insure the policy holder for life as long as the premiums are paid.

Haldol is an antipsychotic medication which is commonly used as a chemical restraint.

Hallucinations are sensory perceptions—sight, taste, sound, etc.—that have no basis in reality. For example, hearing voices telling you to jump off a bridge is an auditory hallucination.

Hemiparesis is one–sided weakness of an arm and leg.

Hemiplegia is one–sided paralysis of an arm and leg.

Hemorrhagic Strokes are cerebrovascular accidents complicated by bleeding into the brain tissue.

Health Maintenance Organization (HMO) is a pre–paid, comprehensive health plan.

Heroic Measures are those aggressive medical procedures which aim to sustain life in a critically ill patient.

Home Health Agency is a private or nonprofit company that delivers skilled nursing service and at least one other therapeutic service to the home.

Homemaker Service is non–medical support in the home for such activities as food preparation, shopping, cleaning and grooming.

Hospice is an organization that provides a dying patient pain relief, emotional support and medical management.

Hydration is fluid given through an intravenous line or feeding tube in a patient unable to drink an adequate amount of liquid.

Hyperglycemia refers to high blood sugar.

Hypertension refers to high blood pressure.

Hypoglycemia refers to low blood sugar.

Hypotension refers to low blood pressure.

Immune System is composed of white blood cells, factors located in the plasma of blood and specific organs. It is the body's defense against infection and foreign substances.

Incontinence is involuntary loss or urine or feces. (See **UI**)

Inflation Rider is that part of an indemnity insurance policy that increases benefits annually in an attempt to keep up with the increase in the consumer price index.

Intermediary (Medicare related) is a private insurance company under contract with the federal government to review and pay Medicare claims to acute care hospitals and nursing homes.

Internist is a physician who has specialized in internal medicine (i.e., the medical care of adults).

Intramuscular (IM) denotes a route of drug administration.

Intravenous (IV)) denotes a route of drug or fluid administration to be given into the blood stream.

Intreavenous Pyelogram (IVP) is a special detailed x–ray examination of the kidneys in which a dye is given to the patient by intravenous injection.

Invasive treatments or procedures involve making an incision or puncture in the skin or inserting an instrument or foreign material into the body.

Ischemic Strokes are caused by a blood clot that lodges in a blood vessel supplying a particular part of the brain which becomes damaged as a result of decreased blood flow.

J. (Jejunostomy) Tube is a type of feeding tube that is inserted through the abdominal into the jejunum (i.e., the second part of the small intestine).

Life Expectancy is the average amount of time that an organism of a given species lives.

Living Will is a document signed by an individual that instructs that they wish to forgo heroic measures.

Longevity is the maximal life expectancy that a species can attain in the absence of disease, predators, environmental privation or accidents. For human beings, longevity is about 85 years.

Long−term Care is a range of medical and support services for individuals who have lost some capacity for self−care due to chronic illness or other conditions and who are expected to need care for some time. Care can be delivered in a medical facility or at home.

LPN stands for licensed practical nurse. An LPN has attended a practical nursing program which stresses clinical nursing skills.

LVN (term used in Texas and California) stands for licensed vocational nurse. (See **LPN**)

Medicaid (Title XIX) is a health care entitlement program 56% of which is funded by the federal government and the balance by state governments.

Medical Record (Chart) is the written documentation of the patient's medical care.

Medicare is a federal health insurance program for people 65 or older that is run by the U.S. Department of Health and Human Services. In Canada it refers to the complete national health program.

Medigap insurance policies, also called Medicare supplements, are private health insurance companies that offer supplemental insurance policies to cover all or part of the Medicare deductibles and co−payment provisions.

Metastasis of cancer refers to the transfer of the diseased cells from one organ to another, non−contiguous organ.

Multi−infarct Dementia is a form of dementia caused by many small strokes.

Myoclonic Jerks in Alzheimer's patients are rapid, jerky movements of the extremities. These are different from seizures.

Naso−gastric Tube (NG Tube) is a feeding tube that is passed through the nose into the stomach.

Nasopharyngeal Aspiration is the process by which a catheter is passed through the nose into that part of the throat which is above the vocal cords (i.e., the nasopharynx) and fluid or secretions are withdrawn by suction.

Nonprofit Facility is one in which earnings are not distributed to anyone.

Nurse Practitioners are registered nurses with advanced training and certification in a specialized field of medicine. They commonly function as physician extenders.

Nursing Assistants (Nurse's Aides) are people who provide the basic care, such as feeding, bathing, etc., to nursing home patients. A nurse's aide cannot give medications or perform nursing treatments.

Nursing Home (Intermediate) is a type of nursing home that contains patients who do not need extensive nursing care. The distinction between intermediate and skilled nursing homes is often arbitrary.

Nursing Home (Skilled) is a health care facility with continuous licensed nurse coverage and which has the capability of providing continuous nursing treatments.

Obstipation is severe constipation.

Occupational Therapists teach patients how to adapt themselves to perform activities of daily living.

Ombudsman (nursing home related) is an individual appointed by a state agency to investigate and mediate patient complaints concerning nursing home care.

Orthostatic Hypotension is a sudden drop in blood pressure usually occurring when a person stands.

Osteoporosis is the age–related process in which defects in formation and maintenance of bone tissue result in overall loss of bone mass. Individuals with osteoporosis are predisposed to fractures.

Otosclerosis refers to hearing loss due to abnormal formation of spongy bone in the inner ear.

Palliative therapies relieve symptoms without curing the disease.

Paranoia (Paranoid) is a mental disorder which can complicate dementia and is characterized by delusions of grandeur and persecution.

Parkinson's Disease is a slowly progressive disorder with a characteristic tremor of resting muscles, slowing of voluntary movements, a shuffling gait, peculiar posture, muscular weakness and a mask-like expression.

Participating Physician is a doctor who agrees to accept assignment of Medicare.

Patient Advocates are patient's family members or friends who serve as their proponent and are closely involved in monitoring their health care.

Patient Care Plan is a written program of care for the patient that identifies the roles of each service in meeting the resident's needs.

PDR stands for *Physician's Desk Reference,* a book published yearly that lists all drugs, their indications, side effects and dosages.

Physical Therapist (PT) is a rehabilitation specialist who works with patients to regain or retain maximal use of specific muscle groups.

PO refers to the oral route of drug administration or food ingestion.

Podiatrist is a college graduate who has four years of additional training at a recognized school of podiatry. Podiatrists can perform treatments or surgeries on the foot.

Posey has become a generic term for physical restraints.

Pneumonia is an infection of the lung.

Presbycusis is age–related deafness due to damage of the auditory nerve.

Pressure Points are those areas of the body must susceptible to decubiti. They are generally located over bony protuberances.

Pressure Ulcers (see Decubiti)

PRN is an abbreviation used on prescriptions denoting "as needed."

Progeria is a genetic disease in which children experience markedly accelerated aging.

Prospective Payment System (PPS) is a Medicare related process started in 1983 under which hospitals are paid fixed amounts based on the principle diagnosis of the patient.

Pseudodementia is a potentially reversible form of confusion. It is characterized by signs and symptoms of depression.

Pulmonary Emphysema is a chronic lung disorder in which lung elasticity is lost.

Reconsideration Unit (Recon) is an intermediary's team, usually composed of medically trained individuals, that reviews rejected Medicare claims on skilled nursing home costs.

Recreational Therapist (RT) is the nursing home's coordinator of recreational activities. All Medicare and Medicaid approved nursing homes must have a qualified RT on staff.

Rehabilitation is the process by which the maximal degree of functional status is restored to a patient.

Report (Nurses' Report) is the exchange of information by the outgoing and incoming nursing shifts. It includes a summary of the status of each patient and a description of any new treatments or change in medication orders.

Resident Council in a nursing home is composed of a group of patients who meet regularly to discuss problems and procedures in a nursing home.

Respirator (Ventilator) is a machine that artificially breathes for the patient.

Rest Home is a custodial facility also known as retirement home, board and care home, enriched housing and other terms.

Restraint (Chemical) is a medication given for the purpose of inhibiting behavior or movement.

Restraint (Physical) is a mechanical appliance used to inhibit movement.

Retirement Village is housing specifically constructed for retired people, 80% of whom must meet minimum age requirements.

RN stands for registered nurse who is a person with specialized scientific and clinical training in nursing skills.

SDAT stands for senile dementia of the Alzheimer's type. (See **Alzheimer's Disease**)

Sedative is a medication given for the purpose of allaying excited behavior or inducing sleep.

Snow (as in "to snow a patient") is the administration of medications to the point at which a patient is semi–conscious. "To snow" is used as a euphemism for "to restrain chemically."

Speech Therapist (ST) is a member of the rehabilitation team who specializes in the treatment of dysfunctional speech and swallowing.

Stroke (See **Cerebrovascular Accident**)

Suction is the aspiration of gas or fluid by mechanical means.

Sundowning refers to nocturnal hyperalertness in a patient with dementia.

Syncope is the sudden loss of consciousness.

Tardive Dyskinesia is a dreaded irreversible complication of antipsychotic therapy marked by rhythmic, jerky movements of the face, mouth or tongue.

Tracheostomy is a surgically made opening through the neck into the windpipe (trachea). A tracheostomy tube ("trach") can be placed through this opening.

Tranquilizer is a drug used to treat anxiety, agitation or neurosis.

Transient Ischemic Attack (TIA) is an episode lasting a few seconds or up to 24 hours and may presage a stroke. Symptoms may include temporary visual disturbance, weakness or tingling of an extremity.

UI stands for urinary incontinence. (See **Incontinence**)

Ultrasound is a type of radiologic test in which sound waves are transmitted through the tissues. A computer generated image is developed by virtue of the velocity of return of the sound waves.

Urinary Tract Infection (UTI) refers to an infection of the urine which may affect any part of the urinary system, including the bladder and the kidneys.

Ventilator (See **Respirator**)

Visiting Nurse is usually a registered nurse who travels to a patient's home to deliver scheduled nursing services.

Walkers are four–legged devices used by individuals who need firm support as they ambulate.

Wanderers are patients with confusion who walk aimlessly.

APPENDIX

STATE AGENCIES ON AGING

If you are unable to contact your local area agency on aging, a nursing home ombudsdman or any other information or service source, it is recommended that you contact your state agency on aging for information.

State	Telephone Number
Alabama Commission on Aging	(205) 242 5743
Older Alaskans Commission	(907) 465 3250
Arizona Office on Aging	(602) 542 4446
Arkansas Department of Human Services	(501) 682 2441
California Department of Aging	(916) 322 3887
Colorado Aging and Adult Services Division	(303) 866 3851
Connecticut Department on Aging	(203) 566 7772
Delaware Division on Aging	(302) 577 4660
District of Columbia Office of Aging	(202) 724 5622
Florida Aging and Adult Services	(904) 488 8922
Georgia Office of Aging	(404) 894 5333
Hawaii Executive Office on Aging	(808) 586 0100
Idaho Office on Aging	(208) 334 3833
Illinois Department of Aging	(217) 785 2870
Indiana Department on Aging	(317) 232 7020
Iowa Commission on Aging	(515) 281 5187
Kansas Department on Aging	(913) 296 4986
Kentucky Division for Aging Services	(502) 564 6930
Louisiana Governor's Office of Elderly Affairs	(504) 925 1700
Maine Bureau of Elderly, Department of Human Services	(207) 624 5335
Maryland Office on Aging	(410) 225 1102
Massachusetts Department of Elder Affairs	(617) 727 7750
Michigan Office of Services to the Aging	(517) 373 8230
Minnesota Board on Aging	(612) 296 2770

State	Telephone Number
Mississippi Council on Aging	(601) 359 6770
Missouri Division of Aging	(314) 751 3082
Montana Community Services Division	(406) 444 3111
Nebraska Department on Aging	(402) 471 2306
Nevada Division for Aging Services	(702) 486 3545
New Hampshire State Council on Aging	(603) 271 4680
New Jersey Division on Aging	(609) 292 0920
New Mexico State Agency on Aging	(505) 827 7640
New York State Office for the Aging	(518) 474 5731
North Carolina Division of Aging	(919) 733 3983
North Dakota Aging Services	(701) 224 2577
Ohio Commission on Aging	(614) 466 1221
Oklahoma Services for the Aging	(405) 521 2327
Oregon Senior Services Division	(503) 378 4728
Pennsylvania Department of Aging	(717) 783 1550
Puerto Rico Gericulture Commission	(809) 722 2429
Rhode Island Department of Elderly Affairs	(401) 277 2858
South Carolina Commission on Aging	(803) 735 0210
South Dakota Office of Adult Services	(605) 773 3656
Tennessee Commission on Aging	(615) 741 2056
Texas Department of Aging	(512) 444 2727
Utah Division of Aging and Adult Services	(801) 538 3910
Vermont Office on Aging	(802) 241 2400
Virginia Department for the Aging	(804) 225 2271
Washington Bureau of Aging and Adult Services	(206) 586 3768
West Virginia Commission on Aging	(304) 558 3317
Wisconsin Office on Aging	(608) 266 2536
Wyoming Commission on Aging	(307) 777 7986

SAMPLE LIVING WILL

To: My Family, Physician, Lawyer

Death is as much a reality as birth, growth, maturity and old age. It is the one certainty of life. If the time comes when I can no longer take part in decisions for my own future, let this statement stand as an expression of my wishes and directions, while I am still of sound mind.

If at such a time the situation should arise in which there is no reasonable expectation of my recovery from extreme physical or mental disability, I direct that I be allowed to die and not be kept alive by medications, artificial means or "heroic measures." I do, however, ask that medication be mercifully administered to me to alleviate suffering even though this may shorten my remaining life.

This statement is made after careful consideration and is in accordance with my strong convictions and beliefs. I want the wishes and directions here expressed carried out to the extent permitted by law. Insofar as they are not legally enforceable, I hope that those to whom this Will is addressed will regard themselves as morally bound by these provisions.

Durable Power of Attorney (optional)

I hereby designate _____to serve as my attorney–in–fact for the purpose of making medical treatment decisions. This power of attorney shall remain in force in the event that I become incompetent or otherwise unable to make such decisions for myself.

Sworn and subscribed to
before me this _____ day
of _____ 19 _____
_____
Notary Public

Signed _____
Date _____
Witness _____
Witness _____

LONG–TERM CARE INSURANCE
BUYER'S CHECKLIST

Feature (Yes/No)	Co. A	Co. B	Co. C
Does the policy pay benefits for skilled, custodial and home care?			
Must you be hospitalized before you receive benefits?			
Does the policy provide coverage for senile dementia?			
Does the company agree to renew as long as premiums are paid?			
Is there an inflation rider?			
Must you have skilled nursing care before you get benefits for custodial or home care?			
Does the plan allow you to choose the amount of daily coverage?			
Will the cost of coverage increase as you get older?			
Will the policy cover you if you move to another area?			
Does the company provide a case manager?			
Will the premium always be based on your age at time of enrollment?			
Is the company qualified to write this insurance in this state?			
What is the waiting period for pre–existing conditions?			

What percentage of the skilled nursing home cost do they pay for:
    Custodial care—
    Home care—			

Feature (Yes/No)	Co. A	Co. B	Co. C

What is their A. M. Best rating?

What is the yearly premium for an $80 a day benefit, with a 90–day waiting period, an inflation rider, for a minimum of two years of coverage?

COMPANIES SELLING LONG–TERM CARE INSURANCE

(as of January 1992)
Company names that are *italicized* are affiliates or subsidiaries of the company above them.

Aetna Life & Casualty[1]
Aid Association for Lutherans[6]
Allstate Life Insurance Company
American Family Life Assurance Company of Columbus
American Independent Insurance Company
American Integrity Insurance Company
American Physicians
American States Life Insurance Company[5]
American Travellers Life Insurance Company
American United Life Insurance Company[5]
AMEX Life Assurance Company
American Centurion Life & Accident Assurance Co.
Anthem Life Insurance Company
Associated Doctors Health and Life Insurance Company
Bankers Life and Casualty Company
Bankers Multiple Line Insurance Company

Certified Life Insurance Company
Union Bankers Insurance Company
Banner Life Insurance Company[5]
Benefit Trust Life Insurance Company
C.S.A. (subsidiary of Blue Cross and Blue Shield of AZ.)
Blue Cross and Blue Shield of Connecticut, Inc.[2]
Hawaii Medical Service Association[2]
Blue Cross and Blue Shield of Indiana
Blue Cross and Blue Shield of Iowa
Blue Cross and Blue Shield of Kansas, Inc.
Blue Cross and Blue Shield of Kansas City
Southeastern United Agency[2] (subsidiary of Blue Cross and Blue Shield of KY)
Blue Cross and Blue Shield of Maryland, Inc.
Blue Cross and Blue Shield of Minnesota[2]
Blue Cross and Blue Shield of Missouri

Blue Cross and Blue Shield of Montana

Blue Cross and Blue Shield of the National Capital Area[2]

Corporate Diversified Services, Inc. (subsidiary of Blue Cross and Blue Shield of NE)

Combined Services, Inc. (subsidiary of Blue Cross and Blue Shield of NH)

Finger Lakes LTC Insurance Company[2] (subsidiary of Blue Cross and Blue Shield of Rochester)

Group Insurance Services (subsidiary of Blue Cross and Blue Shield of NC)

Blue Cross and Blue Shield of North Dakota

Medical Life Insurance Company[2] (subsidiary of Blue Cross/Shield Mutual of Northern OH)

Consumer Services Casualty Insurance Company (subsidiary of Blue Cross of Western Pennsylvania)

Group Services, Inc. (subsidiary of Blue Cross and Blue Shield of UT)

Blue Cross and Blue Shield of Virginia[2]

Blue Cross of Washington and Alaska

King County Medical Blue Shield (Seattle, WA)

Mountain State Blue Cross and Blue Shield (WV)

Blue Cross and Blue Shield of Wyoming

Business Men's Assurance Company[5]

Calfarm Life Insurance Company[5]

Central Life Assurance Company[5]

CIGNA Corporation[1]

Cologne Reinsurance Company[3]

Colonial Life & Accident Insurance Company[6]

Continental Casualty Company (CNA)[2]

Valley Forge Life Insurance Company[5]

Continental General Insurance Company[6]

Continental Western Life Insurance Company[5]

Country Life Insurance Company

Durham Life Insurance Company[5]

Employers Modern Life Insurance Company[5]

Equitable Life and Casualty Company

Equitable Life Insurance Company of Iowa[5]

Farmland Life Insurance Company[5]

Federal Home Life Insurance Company

Harvest Life Insurance Company

First Penn Pacific Life Insurance Company[5]

Georgia Life and Health Insurance Company

Golden Rule Life Insurance Company[5]

Great Fidelity Life Insurance Company

Great Republic Life Insurance Company

Guarantee Mutual Life Insurance Company[5]

Hartford Insurance Company

IDS Life Insurance Company

IDS Life Insurance Company of New York

Independence Nursing Insurance Company

Integrity National Insurance
Company
Interstate Assurance Company[5]
ITT Life Insurance Corporation[5]
J.C. Penney Life Insurance
Company
Jefferson National Life Insurance
Company[5]
John Alden Life Insurance
Company
John Hancock Mutual Life
Insurance Company[2]
Kansas City Life Insurance
Company[5]
Life and Health Insurance Company
of America
Life Investors Insurance Company
of America
*Bankers United Life Assurance
Company[6]*
*Monumental Life Insurance
Company*
PFL Insurance Company[6]
Lincoln Benefit Life Insurance
Company[5]
Lincoln National Life Insurance
Company[6]
Lutheran Brotherhood
Medico Life Insurance Company
*Mutual Protective Insurance
Company*
Metropolitan Life Insurance
Company[7]
Mutual of Omaha[2]
National Travelers Life Company[5]
Nationwide Life Insurance
Company[6]
New York Life Insurance Company
North American Life & Casualty
Company
Northwestern National Life
Insurance Company

Old American Life Insurance
Company
Pan–American Life Insurance
Company[5]
Penn Treaty Insurance Company
Physicians Mutual Insurance
Company
Pilgrim Life Insurance Company
Pioneer Life Insurance Company of
Illinois
The Principal Financial Group[1]
Protected Home Mutual Life
Insurance Company[5]
Provident Life and Accident
Insurance Company
Providers Fidelity Life Insurance
Company
Prudential Insurance Company of
America[2]
Pyramid Life Insurance Company
Security Connecticut Life Insurance
Company
Security Mutual Life Insurance
Company of Lincoln, Nebraska[5]
Sentry Life Insurance Company
Shelter Life Insurance Company[5]
Standard Life & Accident Insurance
Company
State Life Insurance Company of
America[5]
Summit National Life
Teachers Insurance and Annuity
Association[1]
Time Insurance Company[6]
Transamerica Occidental Life
Insurance Company[6]
Transport Life Insurance
The Travelers Insurance Company[7]
United American Insurance
Company
United Farm Bureau Family
Insurance Company[5]

United General Life Insurance Company United Life Insurance Company[5] United Security Assurance Company of Pennsylvania UNUM Life Insurance Company[4] US Life Corporation[5]	*All American Life Insurance Company*[5] *Old American Life Insurance Company*[5] *United States Life Insurance Company of New York*[5]

[1]Provides an employer–sponsored plan.

[2]Provides an individual and employer–sponsored plan.

[3]Provides coverage to members of a continuing care retirement community.

[4]Provides an employer–sponsored plan and coverage to members of a continuing care retirement community.

[5]Offered as part of a life insurance policy.

[6]Provides an individual plan and also offered as part of life insurance policy.

[7]Provides an employer–sponsored plan and also offered as part of life insurance policy.

Sources: Health Insurance Association of America and Blue Cross and Blue Shield Association

Information reprinted courtesy of Health Insurance Association of America.

PATIENT RIGHTS AND RESPONSIBILITIES
SAMPLE PATIENTS' BILL OF RIGHTS

The following principles have been adopted by in accordance with those set forth by the Joint Commission of Accreditation for Hospitals.

1. Any patient admitted shall be informed of his/her rights as a patient in that facility. Evidence by the patient's signature upon a document delineating a patient's rights shall constitute proof that he/she has been informed of all rights, responsibilities, rules and regulations governing patient conduct.
2. Prior to or at the time of admission and during stay, the patient shall be fully informed of the services available at the facility, and related services, including any charges for services not covered under Title XVIII or Title XIX not covered in the basic per diem rate. The patient shall be accorded impartial access to treatment and accommodations.

3. The patient shall have a free choice of physician and be fully informed by his physician of his medical condition unless medically contraindicated, such contraindication to be noted in the medical record. The patient shall be afforded the opportunity to participate in the planning of his medical treatment and to refuse to participate in experimental research. The patient shall be informed of the nature and purpose of any technical procedures that are going to be performed as well as know by whom such procedures are going to be carried out.

4. The patient shall be transferred or discharged only for medical reasons, or for his welfare, or that of other patients, or for non–payment of bills (except as prohibited by Title XVIII or XIX). The patient and his family shall be given reasonable notice of an impending discharge. In an emergency the facility shall have authority to effect immediately a transfer to a facility having more appropriate level of care or services for the patient. Such actions effecting transfer shall be part of the medical record.

5. The patient shall be encouraged and assisted, during his stay to exercise his rights as a citizen: he/she may voice grievances and suggest changes in policy and services of the facility, free from restraint, interference, coercion, discrimination or reprisal.

6. The patient shall be treated so as to be free from mental and physical abuse, and free from chemical and (except in emergencies) physical restraints except as authorized in writing by the attending physician or his designate for a specific and limited period of time.

7. The patient is encouraged to manage his own personal finances and affairs or delegate this responsibility to a person of his choice.

8. The patient shall be assured confidential treatment of his personal and medical record and may approve or refuse the release of information, except in case of transfer to another health care institution or as required by law.

9. The patient shall be treated with dignity and respect at all times; the personal privacy of each patient shall be maintained while providing necessary care.

10. The patient shall not be required to perform services for the facility.

11. The patient may associate and communicate privately with persons of his choice, and may send and receive his personal mail unopened, unless medically contraindicated by his physician and so noted on his medical record.

12. The patient may meet with and participate in activities of social, religious and community groups at his discretion unless medically contraindicated and documented by the physician on the medical record.

13. The patient may retain and use his personal clothing possessions as space permits, unless to do so would infringe upon the right of oth-

ers, unless medically contraindicated and so designated by the physician on the medical record.

14. The patient is assured privacy for visits by his/her spouse; if both are patients in the facility, they will be permitted to share a room unless medically contraindicated and so documented by the attending physician on the medical record.

15. The statement of patient's rights shall be explained to the family and/ or guardian and when the patient has been designated incapable of understanding his her rights the appropriate designated individual or agency shall act on his/her behalf.

16. Patients have the right to review facility inspection reports.

17. Patients may organize, maintain and participate in a patient run resident council as a means of fostering communication between residents and staff, encouraging resident independence and addressing the basic rights of nursing home residents free from administrative interference or reprisal.

18. Patients are entitled to the opinion of two physicians concerning the need for surgery, except in an emergency situation, prior to such surgery being performed.

19. The patient is responsible for providing, to the best of his ability, accurate and complete information about present complaints, past illnesses and hospitalizations, medications and other health related matters; for reporting unexpected changes in his condition to the responsible practitioner; for making it known whether he comprehends a prescribed treatment plan and what is expected of him.

20. The patient is responsible for following the treatment recommended by his primary physician and for following facility rules and regulations affecting patient care and conduct. The patient is responsible for his actions if he refuses treatment or does not follow medical instructions.

21. The patient is responsible for being considerate of the rights of other patients and facility personnel and for his personal behavior in the control of noise, smoking, visitors, etc.

22. The patient is responsible for assuring that the financial obligations of his health care are fulfilled as promptly as possible.

Signature Patient
Signature Guardian/Desg. Agent
Facility Representative

Nursing Home Facts

Percent distribution of nursing home residents by selected functional status. Source National Nursing Home Survey:

Aids Used
Eyeglasses*	63.5%
Hearing aid	6.5

Hearing
Not impaired	78.5%
Partially impaired	16.7
Severely impaired	3.4
Completely lost	.6

Bathing
Independent	11.3%
Requires assistance	88.7

Dressing
Independent	24.6%
Requires assistance	75.4

Eating
Independent	60.7%
Requires assistance	39.3
(Includes tube feeding)	

Mobility
Walks independently	29.3%
Walks with assistance	21.8
Chairfast	39.5
Bedfast	6.5

Transferring
Independent	40.1%
Requires assistance	59.9

Using toilet room
Independent	39.1%
Requires assistance	48.9
Does not use	12.0

Continence
No difficulty	48.1%
Difficulty bowels	1.9
Difficulty bladder	10.3
Difficulty with both	31.7
Ostomy in either	8.1

---

*Eyeglasses might be appropriate in more patients, but they are not used for various reasons.

Percent distribution of nursing home residents by usual living arrangements prior to admission as reported by next of kin. Source National Nursing Home Survey:

Usual living quarters

Own home or apartment	40.8%
Relative's home	20.0
Other private home	3.6
Retirement home, boarding house or rented room	1.7
Another health facility	24.9
Another nursing home	16.6
Acute care hospital	4.9
Mental hospital	2.3

Type of usual living arrangement

Lived alone	26.6%
Lived with spouse	10.4
Lived with spouse and other relatives	1.8
Lived with son or daughter	13.7
Lived with other relatives	8.4
Lived with unrelated persons	3.1
Group living, other nursing home or unknown	30.2

Who lived with resident?

Spouse	12.5%
Children	15.0
Parents	2.0
Sibling	4.2
Grandchildren	6.1
Others	12.3
Non–relative	6.1

BIBLIOGRAPHY

BOOKS

American Psychiatric Association. *Diagnostic and Statistical Manual.* 3rd ed., Washington, D.C.: American Psychiatric Association, 1987.

Bausell, Barker R. *How to Select and Evaluate a Nursing Home.* Beverly, MA: People's Medical Society, 1987.

Braunwald, E.; Isselbacher, K.J.; and Petersdorf, R. G. eds. *Harrison's Principles of Internal Medicine.* New York: McGraw–Hill, 1987.

Butler, Robert N. *Why Survive: Being Old in America.* New York: Harper and Row, 1975.

Caldwell, Esther, and Hegner, Barbara R. *Geriatrics, A Study in Maturity.* Albany, N.Y.: Delmar Publishing, 1981.

Callahan, Daniel. *Setting Limits: Medical Goals in an Aging Society.* New York: Simon and Schuster, 1987.

Commonwealth Fund. *Old, Alone and Poor.* Baltimore, MD: Commonwealth Fund, 1987.

Couper, Donna P. "Aging and Our Families." Thesis. University of CT, 1987.

Finch, C.E., Hayflick, L., eds. *Handbook of Biology of Aging.* 1st ed. New York: Van Nostrand Reinhold Company, 1977.

Finch, C.E., Scheider, E.L., eds. *Handbook of Biology of Aging.* 2d ed. New York: Van Nostrand Reinhold Company, 1985.

Ford Foundation. *The Common Good: Social Welfare and the American Future.* New York: Ford Foundation, 1989.

FRIA (Friends and Relatives of Institutionalized Aged). *A Consumer's Guide to Nursing Home Care in New York State.* New York: FRIA, 1987.

Glaser, B.G., Straus, A.L., *Time for Dying,* Chicago, Aldine, 1968.

Horne, J. *Caregiving: Helping an Aged Loved One.* Chicago, IL: Scott, Foreman and Company, 1985.

Humphrey, Derek and Wickett, Ann. *The Right to Die.* New York: Harper and Row, 1987.

Jenike, M.A. *Handbook of Geriatric Psychopharmacology.* Littleton, MA: PSG Publishing, 1988.

Jones, Rochelle. *The Supermeds*. New York: Charles Scribners, 1988.

Kane, Robert L., and Kane, Rosalie, A. *A Will and a Way—What the United States Can Learn from Canada About Caring for the Elderly*. New York: Columbia University Press, 1985.

Kohn, R.R., ed. *Principles of Mammalian Aging*. 2d ed. Englewood Cliffs, NJ: Prentice–Hall, 1978.

Kraus, Anneta S. *A Guide to Supportive Living Arrangements for Older Citizens*. Wallingford, PA: Geriatric Planning Service, 1984.

Kubler–Ross, Elisabeth. *On Death and Dying*. New York: Macmillian, 1970.

Kunkel, H.G., and Dixon, F.J., eds. *Advances in Immunology*. New York: Academic Press, 1980.

Leshan, Eda. *Oh To Be 50 Again*. New York: Times Books, 1986.

Mace, Nancy L., and Rabins, Peter V. *The 36 Hour Day*. Baltimore, MD: John Hopkins University Press, 1981.

Medawar, Peter. *The Uniqueness of the Individual*. London: Methuen & Co., 1957.

Mendelson, Mary A. *Tender Loving Greed*. New York: Alfred A. Knopf, 1974.

Miller, Benjamin F., and Keane, Clare, eds. *Encyclopedia and Dictionary of Medicine Nursing and Allied Health*. Philadelphia, PA: W.B. Saunders, 1983.

Myers, Edward. *When Patients Die*. New York: Viking, 1986.

Nasif, Janet Z. *The Home Healthcare Solution*. New York: Harper and Row, 1985.

Pieper, Hanns G. *The Nursing Home Primer*. White Hall, VA: Betterway Publications, 1989.

Pifer, Alan and Bronte, Lydia, eds. *Our Aging Society*. New York: W.W. Norton and Company, 1986.

Rhodes, Ann M., and Miller, Robert D. *Nursing and the Law*. Rockville, MD: Aspen Publications, 1984.

Sculty, Thomas. *Playing God, the New World of Medical Choices*. New York: Simon and Schuster, 1987.

Silverstone, Barbara, and Hyman, Helen. *You and Your Aging Parent*. New York: Pantheon Books, 1982.

Skidmore–Roth, Lina. *Mosby's 1989 Drug Reference*. St. Louis, MO: Mosby Co., 1989.

Slater, Harvey. *Pressure Ulcers in the Elderly*. Pittsburg, PA: Synapse Publications, 1988.

Starr, Paul. *Social Transformation of American Medicine*. New York: Basic Books, 1983.

Tantor, Jerry, and Tantor, Mary J. *The Oral Report*. New York: Facts on File, 1988.

Townsend, C.R., and Calon, P., eds. *Physiological Ecology: An Evolutionary Approach to Resource Use*. Oxford. Blackwell, 1981.

Wendland, C. J., and Ouslander, J. G. *A Rehabilitative Approach to Incontinence in Long–Term Care: A Training Manual for Licensed Nurses.* Pasadena, CA: Beverly Foundation, 1986.

Wyngaarden, J.B., and Smith, L.H., eds. *Cecil Textbook of Medicine.* Philadelphia, PA: W.B. Saunders, 1988.

JOURNALS

Applegate, W.B. "Hypertension in Elderly Patients." *Annals of Internal Medicine* **110:** 901–915 (1989).

Avorn, J.; Dreyer, P.; Connelly, K.; et al. "Use of Psychoactive Medication and the Quality of Care in Rest Homes." *New England Journal of Medicine* **320:** 227–232 (1989).

Avorn, J., and Langer E. "Induced Disability in Nursing Home Patients: A Controlled Trial." *Journal of the American Geriatrics Society* **30:** 397–400 (1982).

Baker, S.P., and Harvey, A.H. "Fall Injuries in the Elderly." *Clinical Geriatric Medicine* **1:** 501–512 (1985).

Balin, A.K., and Allen, R.G. "Mechanisms of Biologic Aging." *Dermatology Clinics* **4:** 347–358 (1986).

Bamford, K.A., and Caine, E.D. "Does 'Benign Senescent Forgetfullness' Exist?" *Clinics in Geriatric Medicine* **4:** 897–914 (1988).

Baum H.M. "The National Survey of Stroke: Survival and Prevalence." *Stroke* **12:** 59–68 (1981).

Bedell, S.E.; Delbanco, T.L.; Cook, E.F.; et al. "Survival After Cardiopulmonary Resuscitation in the Hospital." *New England Journal of Medicine* **309:** 569–576 (1983).

Beers, M.; Avorn, J.; Soumerai, S.; and et al. "Psychoactive Medication Use in Intermediate–care Facility Residents." *Journal of the American Association* **260:** 1020 (1988).

Besdine, R.W. "The Maturing of Geriatrics." *New England Journal of Medicine* **320:** 181–182 (1989).

Blazer, D.G. "Depression in the Elderly." *New England Journal of Medicine* **320:** 164–166 (1989).

Blazer, D.G.; Bachar, J. R.; and Manton, K.G. "Suicide in Late Life: Review and Commentary." *Journal of the American Geriatric Society* **34:** 519–525 (1986).

Bloom, M.F. "Dramatic Decrease in Decubitus Ulcers." *Geriatric Nursing.* March/April, 1985. 84–91.

Brandfonbrener, M.; Landowne, M.; and Shock N.W. "Changes in Cardiac Output with Age." *Circulation* **12:** 557–566 (1955).

Budden, F. "Adverse Reactions in Long–term Care Facility Residents. *Journal of the American Geriatrics Society* **33:** 449–450 (1985).

Byyny, R.L. "Hypertension in the Elderly." *The American Journal of Medicine* **81:** 1055–1058 (1986).

Campbell, A.J.; Reinken, J.; Allan, B.C.; et al. "Falls in Old Age: A Study of Frequency and Related Clinical Factors." *Age Ageing* **10:** 264–270 (1981).

Consensus Conference. "Lowering Blood Cholesterol to Prevent Heart Disease." *Journal of the American Medical Association* **253:** 2080–2086 (1985).

DeBusk, F.L. "The Hutchinson-Gilford Progeria Syndrome." *The Journal of Pediatrics* **80:** 697–724 (1972).

Duthie, E.H., and Glatt, S.L. "Understanding and Treating Multi–infarct Dementia." *Clinics in Geriatric Medicine* **4:** 749–766 (1988).

Eckel, F.M., and Crawley, H.K. "A Study of Pharmacy Services in North Carolina Rest Homes." *Journal of the American Pharmaceutical Association* **11:** 387–390 (1971).

Everitt, D.; Learman, L.; and Avorn, J. "Incontinence Related Claims in an Elderly Population." *Gerontologist* **25:** 246–247 (1985).

Fields, W.S. "Multi–infarct Dementia." *Neurology Clinics* **4:** 405–412 (1986).

Fitzgerald, J.F.; Moore, P.S.; and Dittus, R.S. "The Care of Elderly Patients with Hip Fracture: Changes Since Implementation of the Prospective Payment System." *New England Journal of Medicine* **319:** 1392–1397 (1988).

Gleckman, R., and Czachor, J. "Urinary Tract Infections in the Elderly." *Hospital Physician* Dec., 1988: 16–20.

Gurland B., and Toner, J. "The Epidemiology of the Concurrence of Depression and Dementia." In *Alzheimer's Disease: Problems, Prospects, and Perspectives,* ed. H.J. Altman, 45–55. New York: Plenum Press, 1987.

Hayflick, L. "The Aging Process: Current Theories." *Drug–Nutrient Interactions* **4:** 13–33 (1985).

Hayflick, L. "The Cell Biology of Aging." *New England Journal of Medicine* **295:** 1302–1308 (1976).

Hayflick, L., and Moorehead, P.S. "The Serial Cultivation of Human Diploid Cell Strains." *Experimental Cell Research* **25:** 585 (1961).

Herman, J.M. "Present and Future Patterns of Stoke Care." *Clinics in Geriatric Medicine* **2:** 113–119 (1986).

Irvine, P. "An Approach to the Management of Medical Problems in Demented Patients." *Clinics in Geriatric Medicine* **4:** 703–717.

Jacoby, R.J.; Levy, R.; and Dawson, J.M. "Computed Tomography in the Elderly: I. The Normal Population." *British Journal of Psychiatry* **136:** 249–255 (1980).

Jonsson, P.V.; McNamee, M.; and Campion, E.W. "The 'Do Not Resuscitate' Order: A Profile of Its Changing Use.'' *Archives of Internal Medicine* **148:** 2373–2375 (1988).

Kirkwood, T.B.L., and Holliday, F.R.S. ''The Evolution of Aging and Longevity.'' *Proceedings of the Royal Society of London Biology* **205:** 531–546 (1979).

Koller, W.C.; Glatt, S.L.; and Fox, J.H. ''Senile Gait: A Distinct Clinical Entity.'' *Clinical Geriatric Medicine* **1:** 661–669 (1985).

Kosiak, M. ''Etiology and Pathology of Ischemic Ulcers.'' *Archives of Physical Medicine and Rehabilitation* **40:** 62–73 (1959).

Kwentus, J.A.; Hart, R.; Lingon, N.; et al. ''Alzheimer's Disease.'' *The American Journal of Medicine* **81:** 91–95 (1986).

Kynes, P. ''A New Perspective on Pressure Sore Prevention.'' *Journal of Enterostomy Therapeutics* **13:** 173–177 (1986).

Larson, E.B.; Kukull, W.A.; Buchner, D.; et al. ''Diagnostic Tests in the Evaluation of Dementia: A Prospective Study of 200 Elderly Outpatients.'' *Archives of Internal Medicine* **146:** 1917–1922 (1986).

Lavy, S. ''Medical Risk Factors in Stroke.'' *Advance Neurology* **25:** 27–33 (1979).

Lindeman, R.D.; Tobin, J.; and Shock, N.W. ''Longitudinal Studies on the Rate of Decline in Renal Function with Age.'' *Journal of the American Geriatric Society* **33:** 278–285 (1985).

McMenemy, W.H. ''Alois Alzheimer and His Disease.'' In *Alzheimer's Disease and Related Conditions,* eds. Wolstenholme, G.E., and O'Conner, M , 5–9 London: J. & A. Churchill, 1970.

Makinodan, T., and Kay, M.B. ''Age Influence on the Immune System.'' In Advances in Immunology, Volume 29, eds. H.G. Kunkel, and F.J. Dixon, 287–310, New York: Academic Press, 1980.

Maklebust, J. ''Pressure Ulcers: Etiology and Prevention.'' *Nursing Clinics of North America* **22:** 359–376 (1987).

Mann, S.H. ''Practical Management Strategies for Families with Demented Victims.'' *Neurology Clinics* **4:** 469–477 (1986).

Masoro, E.J. ''Biology of Aging, Current State of Knowledge.'' *Archives of Internal Medicine* **147:** 166–169 (1987).

Masoro, E.J. ''Nutrition and Aging: A Current Assessment.'' *Journal of Nutrition* **115:** 842–848 (1985).

Meyer, J.S.; Judd, B.W.; Tawaklna, T.; et al. ''Improved Cognition After Control of Risk Factors for Multi–infarct Dementia.'' *Journal of the American Medical Association* **256:** 2203–2209 (1986).

Morley, J.E. ''Nutritional Status of the Elderly.'' *The American Journal of Medicine* **81:** 679–695 (1986).

Mozar, H.N.; Bal, D.G.; and Howard, J.T. ''Perspectives on the Etiology of Alzheimer's Disease.'' *Journal of the American Medical Association* **257:** 1503–1507 (1987).

Murphy, D.J. "Do-Not-Resuscitate Orders: Time for Reappraisal in Long–term Care Institutions." *Journal of the American Medical Association* **260:** 2098–2101 (1988).

Nevitt, M.C.; Cummings, S.R.; Kidd, S.; et al. "Risk factors for Recurrent Nonsyncopal Falls." *Journal of the American Medical Association* **261:** 2663–2668 (1989).

Ouslander, J.G.; Kane, R.L.; and Abrass, I.B. "Urinary Incontinence in Elderly Nursing Home Patients." *Journal of American Medical Association* **248:** 1194–1195 (1982).

Ouslander, J.G.; Orr, N.K.; Miura, S.A.; et al. "Incontinence Among Dementia Patients: Characteristics, Management and Impact on Caregivers." *Journal of Gerontology* **39:** 453–459 (1988).

Ouslander, J.G.; Uman, G.C.; Urman, H. N.; et al. "Incontinence Among Nursing Home Patients: Clinical and Functional Correlates." *Journal of the American Geriatric Society* **35:** 324–330 (1987).

Polissar, L.; Severson, M.S.; and Brown, N.K. "Factors Affecting Place of Death in Washington State, 1968–1981." *Journal of Community Health* **12:** 40–55 (1987).

Ray W.; Federspiel, C.F.; and Schaffner, W. "A Study of Antipsychotic Drug Use in Nursing Homes: Epidemiologic Evidence Suggesting Misuse." *American Journal of Public Health* **70:** 485–491 (1980).

Resnick, N.M., and Yalla, S.V. "Management of Urinary Incontinence in the Elderly." *New England Journal of Medicine* **313:** 800–805 (1985).

Resnick, N.M.; Yalla, S.V.; and Laurino, E. "The Pathophysiology of Urinary Incontinence Among Institutionalized Elderly Persons." *New England Journal of Medicine* **320:** 1–7 (1989).

Riggs, B.L.; Melton, L.J. "Involutional Osteoporosis." *New England Journal of Medicine* **314:** 1676–1686 (1986).

Robbins, L.J. "Restraining the Elderly." *Clinics in Geriatric Medicine* **2:** 591–599 (1986).

Rodeheffer, R.J.; Gerstenblith, G.; Becker, L.C.; et al. "Exercise Cardiac Output Is Maintained with Advancing Age in Healthy Human Subjects: Cardiac Dilatation and Increased Stroke Volume Compensate for a Diminished Heart Rate." *Circulation* **69:** 203–213 (1984).

Rowe, J.W., and Kahn, R.L. "Human Aging: Usual and Successful." *Science* **237:** 143–149 (1987).

Sager, M.A.; Easterling, D.V.; Kindig, D.A.; et al. "Changes in the Location of Death After Passage of Medicare's Prospective Payment System: A National Study." *New England Journal of Medicine* **320:** 433–439 (1989).

Schiedermayer, D.L. "The Decision to Forgo CPR in the Elderly Patient." *The Journal of the American Medical Association* **260:** 2096–2097 (1988).

Schuchmann, J. "Stoke Rehabilitation." *Postgraduate Medicine* **74:** 101–111 (1983).

Schut, L.J. "Dementia Following Stroke." *Clinics in Geriatric Medicine* **4:** 767–780 (1988).

Siegel, B.; Gershon, S. "Dementia, Depression, and Pseudodementia." In *Alzheimer's Disease: Problems, Prospects, and Perspectives*, ed. H.J. Altman, New York: Plenum Press, 1987.

Sier, H.; Ouslander, J., and Orzeck, S. "Urinary Incontinence Among Geriatric Patients in an Acute-care Hospital." *Journal of the American Medical Association* **257:** 1767–1771 (1987).

Silliman, R.A.; Wagner, E.H.; and Fletcher, R.H. "The Social and Functional Consequences of Stroke for Elderly Patients." *Stroke* **18:** 200–203 (1987).

Smith, G.S., and Walford, R.L. "Influence of the Main Histocompatibility Complex on Aging in Mice." *Nature:* **270:** 727 (1977).

Taffet, G.E.; Teasdale, T.A.; and Luchi, R.J. "In-hospital Cardiopulmonary Resuscitation." *Journal of the American Medical Association* **260:** 2069–2072 (1988).

Tinetti, M.E. "Factors Associated with Serious Injury During Falls by Ambulatory Nursing Home Residents." *Journal of the American Geriatric Society* **35:** 644–648 (1987).

Tinetti, M.E., and Speechley, M. "Prevention of Falls Among the Elderly." *New England Journal of Medicine* **320:** 1055–1059 (1989).

Tomlinson, Tom, and Brody, H. "Ethics and Communication in Do–Not–Resuscitate Orders." *New England Journal of Medicine* **318:** 43–46 (1986).

Uhlmann, R.F.; Larson, E.B.; Rees, T.S.; et al. "Relationship of Hearing Impairment to Dementia and Cognitive Dysfunction in Older Adults." *Journal of the American Medicine Association* **261:** 1916–1920 (1989).

Vetter, N.J.; Jones, D.A.; and Victor, D.A. "Urinary Incontinence in Elderly Nursing Home Patients." *Lancet* **2:** 1275–1277 (1981).

Walford, R.L., et al. "The Immunopathology of Aging." In *Annual Review of Gerontology and Geriatrics*, Volume 2, eds. C. Eisdorfer, B. Starr, and V. Cristofalo, 215–257. New York: Springer, 1981.

Wells, C.E. "Pseudodementia." *American Journal of Psychiatry* **136:** 895–900 (1979).

Williams, G.C. "Pleiotropy, Natural Selection, and the Evolution of Senescence." *Evolution* **11:** 398–411 (1957).

Williams, M.E., and Pannill, F.C. "Urinary Incontinence in the Elderly. *Annals of Internal Medicine* **97:** 895–907 (1982).

Wylie, C.M. "The Value of Early Rehabilitation in Stroke." *Geriatrics* **25:** 107–113 (1970).

INDEX

ABOUT THE AUTHORS

Mary Brumby Forrest, L.P.N., is a charge nurse at a Connecticut convalescent hospital.

Christopher Forrest, M.D., graduated from the Boston University School of Medicine and completed his residency at the University of Pennsylvania in Philadelphia. He is presently continuing his post–doctoral work in public health issues at Johns Hopkins Medical Center.

Richard Forrest attended the University of South Carolina and the Dramatic Workshop in New York City. He worked in the insurance industry for a number of years until he resigned his position as vice president of a major company to become a full–time writer. He has published fifteen mystery and suspense novels and is also the author of *Alternative Housing for the Elderly*.